T0264241

Updates in Implants for Foot and Ankle Surgery: 35 Years of Clinical Perspectives

Editor

MEAGAN M. JENNINGS

CLINICS IN PODIATRIC MEDICINE AND SURGERY

www.podiatric.theclinics.com

Consulting Editor
THOMAS J. CHANG

October 2019 • Volume 36 • Number 4

ELSEVIER

1600 John F. Kennedy Boulevard • Suite 1800 • Philadelphia, Pennsylvania, 19103-2899

http://www.theclinics.com

CLINICS IN PODIATRIC MEDICINE AND SURGERY Volume 36, Number 4
October 2019 ISSN 0891-8422, ISBN-13: 978-0-323-70928-6

Editor: Lauren Boyle
Developmental Editor: Laura Kavanaugh

Clinics in Podiatric Medicine and Surgery (ISSN 0891-8422) is published quarterly by Elsevier Inc., 360 Park Avenue South, New York, NY 10010-1710. Months of issue are January, April, July, and October. Business and Editorial Offices: 1600 John F. Kennedy Blvd., Ste. 1800, Philadelphia, PA 19103-2899. Customer Service Office: 3251 Riverport Lane, Maryland Heights, MO 63043. Periodicals postage paid at New York, NY and additional mailing offices. Subscription prices are $304.00 per year for US individuals, $574.00 per year for US institutions, $100.00 per year for US students and residents, $382.00 per year for Canadian individuals, $693.00 for Canadian institutions, $439.00 for international individuals, $693.00 per year for international institutions and $220.00 per year for Canadian and foreign students/residents. To receive student/resident rate, orders must be accompanied by name of affiliated institution, date of term, and the *signature* of program/residency co-ordinator on institution letterhead. Orders will be billed at individual rate until proof of status is received. Foreign air speed delivery is included in all *Clinics* subscription prices. All prices are subject to change without notice. POSTMASTER: Send address changes to *Clinics in Podiatric Medicine and Surgery*, Elsevier Health Sciences Division, Subscription Customer Service, 3251 Riverport Lane, Maryland Heights, MO 63043. **Customer Service: 1-800-654-2452 (US). From outside of the US, call 314-447-8871. Fax: 314-447-8029. E-mail: JournalsCustomerService-usa@elsevier.com (for print support); JournalsOnlineSupport-usa@elsevier.com (for online support).**

Reprints. For copies of 100 or more of articles in this publication, please contact the Commercial Reprints Department, Elsevier Inc., 360 Park Avenue South, New York, NY 10010-1710. Tel.: 212-633-3874; Fax: 212-633-3820; E-mail: reprints@elsevier.com.

Clinics in Podiatric Medicine and Surgery is covered in *MEDLINE/PubMed (Index Medicus)* and *EMBASE/Excerpta Medica.*

Contributors

CONSULTING EDITOR

THOMAS J. CHANG, DPM
Clinical Professor and Past Chairman, Department of Podiatric Surgery, California College of Podiatric Medicine, Faculty, The Podiatry Institute, Redwood Orthopedic Surgery Associates, Santa Rosa, California

EDITOR

MEAGAN M. JENNINGS, DPM, FACFAS
Attending, Silicon Valley Foot and Ankle Reconstructive Surgery Fellowship, Staff Surgeon, Palo Alto Medical Foundation, Mountain View, California

AUTHORS

KENDALL ANIGIAN, MD
Department of Orthopaedic Surgery, UT Southwestern Medical Center, Dallas, Texas

GEORGEANNE BOTEK, DPM, FACFAS
Staff, Orthopedic Surgery, Cleveland Clinic, Cleveland, Ohio

MELINDA A. BOWLBY, DPM, AACFAS
Attending Surgeon, Department of Orthopedics, Division of Podiatry, Swedish Medical Center, Seattle, Washington; Attending Surgeon, Department of Orthopedics, Division of Podiatry, Providence Medical Center, Private Practice, The Ankle and Foot Clinic of Everett, Everett, Washington

BRITTANY A. BROWER, DPM
Third Year Chief Foot and Ankle Surgery Resident Physician, John Peter Smith Hospital, Fort Worth, Texas

MICHELLE L. BUTTERWORTH, DPM, FACFAS
Foot and Ankle Physician, Chief of Medical Staff, Williamsburg Regional Hospital, Kingstree, South Carolina

MARY E. CRAWFORD, DPM, FACFAS
Attending Surgeon, Department of Orthopedics, Division of Podiatry, Staff Foot and Ankle Physician, Providence Regional Medical Center, Private Practice, The Ankle and Foot Clinic of Everett, Everett, Washington

THANH DINH, DPM, FACFAS
Program Director, Podiatric Surgical Residency Program, Assistant Professor, Department of Surgery, Division of Podiatry, Beth Israel Deaconess Medical Center, Harvard Medical School, Boston, Massachusetts

KATHERINE E. DUX, DPM, FACFAS
Assistant Professor, Department of Orthopedic Surgery and Rehabilitation, Section of Podiatric Surgery, Loyola University Chicago, Stritch School of Medicine, Maywood, Illinois

DENA EL-SAYED, MD
Internal Medicine Clinic, Infectious Diseases Clinic, Ventura County Medical Center, Ventura, California

SAMANTHA FIGAS, DPM
PGY-2, Resident, Podiatry, Mercy Health Regional Medical Center, Lorain, Ohio

MEAGAN M. JENNINGS, DPM, FACFAS
Attending, Silicon Valley Foot and Ankle Reconstructive Surgery Fellowship, Staff Surgeon, Palo Alto Medical Foundation, Mountain View, California

JACLYN KAPILOW, MD
Department of Orthopaedic Surgery, UT Southwestern Medical Center, Dallas, Texas

CASEY LEWIS, DPM
PGY-2, Department of Surgery, Division of Podiatry, Beth Israel Deaconess Medical Center, Harvard Medical School, Boston, Massachusetts

VICTORIA LIEW, BS
California College of Podiatric Medicine, Samuel Merritt University, Oakland, California

BREANA MARINE, BS
California College of Podiatric Medicine, Samuel Merritt University, Oakland, California

ROYA MIRMIRAN, DPM, FACFAS
Sutter Medical Group, Sacramento, California

SAI NARRA, DPM
PGY-1, Resident, Podiatry, Mercy Health Regional Medical Center, Lorain, Ohio

AKSONE NOUVONG, DPM, FACFAS
Health Sciences Clinical Professor, Department of Surgery, Division of Vascular Surgery, David Geffen School of Medicine at UCLA, Los Angeles, California

KATHERINE M. RASPOVIC, DPM, FACFAS
Assistant Professor, Department of Orthopaedic Surgery, UT Southwestern Medical Center, Dallas, Texas

HANNAH SAHLI, DPM
Resident, Department of Podiatric Surgery, Advent Health System, Orlando, Florida

AMBER SHANE, DPM, FACFAS
Chair, Department of Podiatric Surgery, Faculty, Advent East Podiatric Surgical Residency, Advent Health System, Orlando Foot and Ankle Clinic, Orlando, Florida

BREANN TISANO, MD
Department of Orthopaedic Surgery, UT Southwestern Medical Center, Dallas, Texas

MARIA UGRINICH, DPM
Attending Physician, Penn Presbyterian Medical Center, Philadelphia, Pennsylvania

TRACEY C. VLAHOVIC, DPM, FFPM, RCPS (Glasg)
Clinical Professor, Department of Podiatric Medicine, Temple University School of Podiatric Medicine, Philadelphia, Pennsylvania

TENAYA A. WEST, DPM
Chief Surgical Resident, Kaiser San Francisco Bay Area Foot and Ankle Residency Program, Department of Orthopedics and Podiatric Surgery, Kaiser Foundation Hospitals, Oakland, California

MITZI L. WILLIAMS, DPM, FACFAS, FACFAP
Professor and Attending Surgeon, Kaiser San Francisco Bay Area Foot and Ankle Residency Program, Department of Orthopedics and Podiatric Surgery, Oakland, California

MELISSA YOUNGER, DPM, AACFAS
Independence Foot and Ankle Associates, LLC, Perkasie, Pennsylvania

Contents

> There are a variety of materials available for surgical reconstruction of the foot and ankle. The material that provides the best physical properties to match the mechanical stress should be chosen. Ideal implant material should be biocompatible, nontoxic, noncarcinogenic, nonpyrogenic, and nonallergenic. Key properties include strength, durability, and resistance to fatigue. The material should have ductility to provide continued strength once it has been adapted to the bone surface. The material should be readily available, affordable, and reproducible. Materials that are available for use are stainless steel, cobalt chrome alloys, titanium and titanium alloys, pyrolytic carbon, thermoplastics, and bioceramics.

> Tendinopathy is a common but disabling condition. The term describes a complex, multifaceted pathology of the tendon characterized by pain, decreased function, and reduced exercise tolerance. Tendinopathy accounts for up to 30% of general practice musculoskeletal consultations. Advances in understanding the disease process include inflammation as part of the early tendinopathy process. Once thought to not contribute to the early process of tendon degeneration, this hypothesis has been refuted. This allows guidance in conservative treatment. However, when conservative treatments fail, there are minimally invasive injections and ultrasonic debridement techniques that offer an intermediate treatment step with low reported morbidity.

> Flexible fixation has been described and utilized in various aspects of foot and ankle surgery over the past several decades. In regards to ankle surgery, flexible fixation devices have been used for stabilization of the ankle syndesmosis and augmentation of lateral collateral ankle ligament repair.

In the foot, flexible fixation devices have been incorporated into hallux valgus or varus correction, Lisfranc injury repair, and more recently spring ligament repair augmentation. This article reviews the various applications for flexible fixation in foot and ankle surgery, as well as evidence-based literature on surgical applications and clinical outcomes.

Amnion and chorion products show great promise and have real potential to be mainstays of treatment for chronic, nonhealing wounds. Although amniotic products do carry a cost, the decrease in time to healing, with the assumed subsequent decrease in complication and infection rates, should also be taken into consideration. These products, with their unique biologic potential and availability in the clinical setting, may prove to be beneficial in a vast array of podiatric surgical applications.

Evidence-based medicine continues to guide our treatment of patients. Owing to the unique characteristics of the first metatarsophalangeal joint (1st MTPJ) with its small surface area and the significant amount of multiplanar force that affects it, finding the perfect implant to allow motion and alleviate pain is still the ultimate goal. While some of the older metallic implants and silastic spacers may still be providing pain relief and function to patients, the majority have failed and caused significant bone loss along the way. The HemiCap implants have shown some promise in select patients and may still be a viable option in patients desiring maintenance of 1st MTPJ motion.

Total ankle arthroplasty has been in development for more than 40 years. Although early designs were experimental with high failure rates, current implants are significantly improved, showing promising functional results and clinical outcomes. Total ankle replacement designs are split into mobile-bearing and fixed-bearing designs. When deciding whether to perform ankle arthroplasty, many factors need to be considered to determine if the patient is suitable and which implant is the best fit for patient and surgeon. Many prostheses are available in the United States today and the purpose of this article is to outline options for foot and ankle surgeons.

Use of orthobiologics in sports medicine and musculoskeletal surgery has gained significant interest. However, many of the commercially available and advertised products are lacking in clinical evidence. Widespread use of products before fully understanding their true indications may result in unknown adverse outcomes and may also lead to increased health care costs. As more products become available, it is important to remain judicial in use and to practice evidence-based medicine. Likewise, it is important to continue advances in research in hopes to improve surgical outcomes. This article reviews clinical evidence behind common orthobiologics in the treatment of foot and ankle pathology.

Dena El-Sayed and Aksone Nouvong

Infection can be a devastating complication of surgically inserted prosthetic implants and intramedullary rods, plates and pins. About 2 million implants were inserted in the United States in 2004, and, despite appropriate perioperative antibiotics, approximately 5% of internal fixation devices became infected. Infection rates in fractures that pierce the skin can be as high as 22.7%. Complications of infection include excessive antibiotic use, implant removal, reoperation, and potential amputation. Infections caused by colonized prosthetic implants are often difficult to predict, diagnose, and treat, because they form biofilms. This article explores the approach to infected implants.

Roya Mirmiran and Melissa Younger

Lesser digit deformities that require surgical intervention may be corrected by interphalangeal arthrodesis. The traditional fixation device used to stabilize an interphalangeal arthrodesis is a smooth Kirschner wire (K-wire). Its use, however, has been associated with risks. The K-wires are known to migrate and break, and there are increased risks of pin tract infection. Choices for digital implants include nonresorbable, resorbable, and allograft. There are more than 60 newer intramedullary fixation devices available for use in digital surgery. Intramedullary implants also have their own inherent risks. Further research into patient outcomes and cost-effectiveness of these new devices is still needed.

Georgeanne Botek, Samantha Figas, and Sai Narra

Understanding new theories of the epidemiology of Charcot neuroarthropathy is practice changing. Treatment of Charcot neuroarthropathy is evolving from a passive approach to one that sees the urgency of proactive, early recognition, thereby avoiding the cascading events that lead to the complex, limb-threatening deformities. Preventive medicine is the most efficient at avoiding severe deformity, with prolonged offloading and immobilization as the current mainstay of treatment. However, with recent advancements in medical and surgical modalities, this may become the treatment of the past as clinicians begin to favor medical management and early surgical intervention.

Tracey C. Vlahovic

The lower extremity presents several challenges from a dermatologic standpoint: there are different anatomic areas that not only vary from a stratum corneum thickness and histologic standpoint but are also subject to trauma that is unique (shoe gear, gait cycle). Attention to appropriate diagnosis and management is always warranted but should be especially vigilant to those treating issues of the lower extremity. This article reviews diagnosis and treatment of the most common skin and nail conditions of the foot and ankle.

Opioid Crisis and Acute Pain Management After Foot and Ankle Surgery   695

Melinda A. Bowlby and Mary E. Crawford

Opioid abuse has plagued the United States, with a resurgence since the early 2000s. Governmental agencies, pharmaceutical companies, patients, and physicians have all contributed to this crisis. Severe pain has been reported following foot and ankle surgery. There are current national guidelines for chronic opioid prescribing, but guidelines for acute pain have not been established. Prescribing fewer opioids, education on opioid risks, proper disposal of unused medication, and participating in prescription monitoring programs help reduce opioid abuse. Multimodal analgesia is paramount in managing pain while reducing opioid consumption after postoperative foot and ankle surgery.

Women in Podiatry and Medicine   707

Brittany A. Brower, Meagan M. Jennings, Michelle L. Butterworth, and Mary E. Crawford

The role of female physicians has advanced among western medicine. Women now constitute a majority within medical schools, and the number of women in podiatric medicine and surgery has increased over the last 5 decades. Conversely, female physicians continue to face barriers to closing the gender gap. They have lower academic standings and fewer publications, receive less awards/grants, are underrepresented in leadership positions, have a lower incidence pursuing surgical specialties, and receive lower compensation. Women experience an increased rate of burnout, gender discrimination, and sexual harassment. Increasing awareness of the gender gap is vital to the enhancement of the medical community.

CLINICS IN PODIATRIC MEDICINE AND SURGERY

FORTHCOMING ISSUES

January 2020
Biomechanics of the Lower Extremity
Jarrod Shapiro, *Editor*

April 2020
Top Research in Podiatry Education
Thomas Chang, *Editor*

RECENT ISSUES

July 2019
Diabetes
Paul Jeong Kim, *Editor*

April 2019
Current Perspectives on Management of
Calcaneal Fractures
Thomas S. Roukis, *Editor*

SERIES OF RELATED INTEREST

Foot and Ankle Clinics
Available at: www.foot.theclinics.com
Orthopedic Clinics
Available at: www.orthopedic.theclinics.com

THE CLINICS ARE AVAILABLE ONLINE!
Access your subscription at:
www.theclinics.com

Dedication

In Memoriam

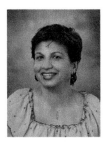

Aprajita Nakra, DPM, FACFAS
(1971–2019)

Aprajita Nakra, DPM, FACFAS was a true role model for female physicians, but her passion for education and teaching made her a true leader and trailblazer for our entire podiatric profession. She was a dedicated physician and skilled foot and ankle surgeon whose innovative energy has helped move our profession forward and remain on the cutting edge of medicine and surgery. She was truly one of the top women in our profession, and she led by example. She graduated from the New York College of Podiatric Medicine in 1997 and then completed a 3-year surgical residency at Emory Northlake Regional Medical Center in 2000. Her thirst for knowledge and her true leadership skills then awarded her numerous accolades and accomplishments. Her successes are many, but there are some highlights that deserve attention.

Dr Nakra's inspiring career included becoming board certified in foot and recon-structive rearfoot and ankle surgery as well as becoming certified in many different total ankle replacement systems. She served as a President of the Arizona Podiatric Medical Society and was the first female President of the Arizona State Physicians' Association. She founded Advanced Ankle and Foot in Gilbert, Arizona in 2004 and was the Chief Medical Officer of Elite Experts. She was a residency director of the Arizona Division of St. John's Episcopal Hospital and an active faculty member of the Midwestern University Arizona School of Podiatric Medicine.

Dr Nakra was also an active member of the Podiatry Institute, where she chaired many annual conferences as well as lectured extensively domestically as well as inter-nationally. She authored textbook chapters and journal articles and served as a coed-itor of *McGlamry's Comprehensive Textbook of Foot and Ankle Surgery*, fourth edition. Aprajita's altruistic spirit also led her to partake in many medical missions from Central and South America to Africa and Southeast Asia.

Let's continue down Dr Nakra's prestigious path and make her proud! Let's continue to support and encourage one another. Let's assist each other not only in the realm of medicine but also in everyday life. Let's push the bar and continue to make a difference

Clin Podiatr Med Surg 36 (2019) xiii–xiv
https://doi.org/10.1016/j.cpm.2019.07.006
0891-8422/19/© 2019 Published by Elsevier Inc.

podiatric.theclinics.com

for our patients and our profession. Simply put, let's continue to pay it forward like Aprajita always did in every aspect of her life.

It is a true honor, and I am humbled to share some professional accomplishments on behalf of this phenomenal physician and woman. My heart is heavy, but my spirit is high when I reflect on the life and career of Dr Aprajita Nakra. She has touched the lives of so many and will be sorely missed. I have shared with you some of her many great achievements throughout her illustrious career, but what I will miss most is her "never-quit-and-fight-until-the-end" attitude, her endearing nature, her endless compassion, and her true support and friendship. Our profession has lost a great physician, and we have lost an amazing woman, but her legacy will live on through us. There has been a scholarship fund created in the memory of Dr Aprajita Nakra. It will aid in funding female residents to attend the Podiatry Institute's annual "Women's Conference." Details can be found on the Podiatry Institute Web site.

In deep gratitude and appreciation for a truly remarkable woman,

Michelle L. Butterworth, DPM, FACFAS
Williamsburg Regional Hospital
500 Thurgood Marshall Hwy, Suite B
Kingstree, SC 29556, USA

E-mail address:
mbutter@ftc-i.net

Foreword

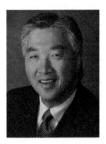

Thomas J. Chang, DPM
Consulting Editor

It is with excitement we present this issue to all foot and ankle surgeons around the world. It is even more exciting this issue is solely written by an extremely talented list of female educators who have come together to share their knowledge on foot and ankle fixation. On the heels of the US Women's World Cup victory and dialogue on parity in salary, we live in a world where there is still a noticeable gender difference in relevant areas of professional and academic achievements. Salaries in general are still lower among female physicians as well as numbers in academic appointments, articles published, and accolades awarded. This is well described in Dr Brower and colleagues' article within this issue.

As many of us in medicine, we are often blessed with significant role models who have helped to shape us into the physicians we are today. I am also blessed to have the guidance of strong women role models in my life. My mom raised 4 young kids on her own. While I was a student at Temple University, I also remember the impact of female role models. Dr Mary Crawford was a few years ahead of me, and our senior year "Professor of the Year" was Dr Jane Pontious. I was surrounded by exceptional and talented male and female residents in my training and have had the privilege of training both men and women in our field over the years. Parity on all levels of professional and academic circles will arrive quicker when more female role models and leaders emerge and are recognized in their communities and nationally.

Dr Meagan Jennings has done a stellar job of bringing together nationally recognized female educators in Podiatric Medicine and Surgery. Although it really should not be necessary to dedicate this issue to Women in Education, we feel it is timely, and continues the conversation of spotlighting the important and evolving role that women play in a traditionally male-dominated profession. I hope this issue highlights the

Clin Podiatr Med Surg 36 (2019) xv–xvi
https://doi.org/10.1016/j.cpm.2019.07.005
0891-8422/19/© 2019 Published by Elsevier Inc.

podiatric.theclinics.com

tremendous contributions these female authors have made to this profession and affirms the fact that quality education is not based on gender.

Thomas J. Chang, DPM
Redwood Orthopedic Surgery Associates
208 Concourse Boulevard
Santa Rosa, CA 95403, USA

E-mail address:
thomaschang14@comcast.net

Preface

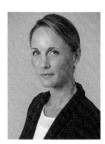

Meagan M. Jennings, DPM, FACFAS
Editor

> *I was taught that the way of progress was neither swift nor easy.*
> —*Marie Curie, physicist, chemist, and winner of the 1903 Nobel Prize in Physics and the 1911 Nobel Prize in Physics.*

While we have made great strides as a profession, the evolution of our profession has not been "swift or easy." That being said, I am honored to be asked to guest edit one of the 35th Anniversary issues of *Clinics in Podiatric Medicine and Surgery*. When reviewing the Preface and Table of Contents of Volume 1, Number 1 from April 1984, it struck me how far we as podiatric physicians and surgeons have come. The inaugural issue was guest edited by Lowell Scott Weil, DPM and focused on implants. In his Preface, he stated, "…more than 25 implants have been developed for use in foot surgery." Just think about that statement for a second, and I think you will agree that we have advanced as a profession remarkably well over the past 35 years. However, it has not been "swift or easy." We now have hundreds of different foot AND ankle implants, not just foot implants. I applaud the groundwork Dr Weil laid as well as many others to help us advance our profession, our scope of practice, our relationships with engineering and industry, and our integration into every medical community.

The second thing that struck me when reviewing the original *Clinics in Podiatry Medicine and Surgery* was that all but 2 (out of 24) authors were men. Thirty-five years ago, the female presence in podiatry was not nearly what it is today. Today, almost 50% of our Colleges of Podiatric Medicine and Surgery are women. Kristy Weber, MD recently stated upon induction as American Academy of Orthopedic Surgeons president, "While my gender does not define me, I know that reducing barriers and embracing gender, ethnic and racial diversity in our field only stands to better our culture and better serve patients. By incorporating our unique experiences and perspectives, we can care for a more diverse patient population." I couldn't agree more. This special issue is composed of all female authors and clearly demonstrates the contributions these physicians have made to podiatry and the advancement of our profession. The podiatric profession has made significant progress, and we shall continue to do so

Clin Podiatr Med Surg 36 (2019) xvii–xviii
https://doi.org/10.1016/j.cpm.2019.07.004
0891-8422/19/© 2019 Published by Elsevier Inc.

podiatric.theclinics.com

with open minds and collaboration among ourselves as well as the entire medical community.

Meagan M. Jennings, DPM, FACFAS
Silicon Valley Foot and Ankle Reconstructive Surgery Fellowship
Palo Alto Medical Foundation
701 E. El Camino Real South Wing
Mountain View, CA 94040, USA

E-mail address:
mmjfootankle@gmail.com

Implantable Materials Update

Katherine E. Dux, DPM

KEYWORDS

- Implant materials • Foot and ankle surgery • Metallic implants • Pyrolytic carbon
- Thermoplastics • Bioceramics

KEY POINTS

- Understanding the basic concepts and characteristics of the available implant materials is important for surgical success and optimal patient satisfaction.
- The physical properties of the implant material need to match the mechanical stress applied to the implant, or failure of the device may occur.
- The key properties of an implant material include strength, durability, and resistance to fatigue. The material should be readily available, affordable, and reproducible.
- Current materials that are available for use are stainless steel, cobalt-chrome alloys, titanium and titanium alloys, pyrolytic carbon, thermoplastics, and bioceramics.

Implant materials are commonly used devices in foot and ankle surgery. They function to provide internal stability to osseous and tendinous structures. They are an essential component in many reconstructive procedures of the foot and ankle. The physical properties of the materials need to match the mechanical stress applied to the implant, or failure of the device may occur. They are placed in direct contact with viable tissues and body fluids, which can create a potentially reactive situation both macroscopically and microscopically. Understanding the basic concepts and characteristics of the materials is important for surgical success. Ideal implant material should be biocompatible, nontoxic, noncarcinogenic, nonpyrogenic, and nonallergenic. The key properties of an implant material include strength, durability, and resistance to fatigue. The material should have ductility in order to provide continued strength once it has been adapted to the bone surface. Low-stress relaxation is essential for metallic implants, as this is necessary to maintain compression. The material should be readily available, affordable, and reproducible. Materials that are available for use are stainless steel, cobalt-chrome alloys, titanium and titanium alloys, pyrolytic carbon, thermoplastics, and bioceramics.

Disclosure Statement: The author has nothing to disclose.
Department of Orthopedic Surgery and Rehabilitation, Section of Podiatric Surgery, Loyola University Chicago, Stritch School of Medicine, 2160 South First Avenue, Maywood, IL 60153, USA
E-mail address: Kdux1@lumc.edu

Clin Podiatr Med Surg 36 (2019) 535–542
https://doi.org/10.1016/j.cpm.2019.06.001
0891-8422/19/© 2019 Elsevier Inc. All rights reserved.

METALLIC IMPLANT MATERIALS
Surgical Stainless Steel

Surgical stainless steel (316LVM) contains iron, chromium, nickel, molybdenum, and a very small amount of carbon. Several types of stainless steel are available, and the most widely used for implant manufacture is austenitic stainless steel. To be austenitic at room temperature, stainless steel needs to contain a certain amount of austenite stabilizing elements, such as nickel or molybdenum. Each of the alloy components is added to create a certain effect within the steel, for improved stability or greater fatigue resistance. Stainless steel is hardened by cold working for improved strength and hardness.[1]

The current modification of stainless steel that is used and has proved the most functional is 316 LVM. It is recommended by the American Society of Testing and Materials. L stands for "low" carbon and VM stands for "vacuum remelting."[1] Both modifications make the stainless steel a more ideal material. A lower level of carbon reduces corrosion of the implant within body tissues. Vacuum remelting aids in reducing the metals impurities and improves the flaws within the metal by reducing the amount of bubbles. The 316 steel can be machined, which allows for control of the mechanical properties of the steel.

AISI 316 (American Iron and Steel Institute) LVM stainless steel, when applied within human tissues, demonstrates minimal reaction with a layer of oxidation that provides protection to some forms of corrosion. There is an absence of detrimental intramuscular changes. Pseudomembrane formation is a natural sequela, and this fibrous capsule contains no acute inflammatory foci. This group of stainless steel may still corrode within the body, and is more likely to occur in areas that lack oxygen, such as screw-plate interface or in high-stress areas. This is best described as a zone of chronic inflammation, and fibrosis can be seen between the cortical bone and implant.[2] The tissue adjacent to the implant shows macrophages with iron deposits and foreign body giant cells on a histologic level. This process is more benign with newer implant metals; however, older metals create a substantial fibrotic capsule with more corrosion products and inflammatory cells.[3]

Stainless steel has the potential to create allergic reactions due to its composition of different metals. Nickel has been identified as the most common element responsible for an allergic reaction. It has been demonstrated to cause eczematous dermatitis. Nickel can leach from the implant and cross cell membranes, altering cell function. Malignant degeneration of tissue has been documented due to nickel.[1]

Cobalt-Chromium–Based Alloys

These alloys contain a combination of cobalt, chromium, molybdenum, and carbon. They do not contain nickel. This alloy is used in the manufacturing of artificial joints, and is not used for internal fixation. This metal does not provide the best bone integration properties. Cobalt has a history of toxic effects. Heath and colleagues,[4] in 1971, demonstrated wear particles from total joint prosthesis in rat models made of cobalt-chromium-molybdenum, which led to the development of sarcomata. The disadvantages of using cobalt-chrome alloys as implantable materials may be minimized through techniques that coat the surface of the implant with titanium, at the contact area with bone.[2]

Titanium and Titanium Alloys

Titanium is very lightweight due to its low specific gravity. This makes it a desirable metal for implant fabrication, in addition to its ability to resist corrosion. Titanium has the ability to integrate within the surrounding bone after implanted. Titanium in its elementally pure form is very soft and ductile. The addition of alloying elements, such as aluminum and vanadium, increase the strength of titanium, but reduce some of the ductility. The titanium alloy Ti6Al4V is primarily used in the construction of implants.

The reduced workability of titanium is one negative effect of the addition of alloying metals. Vanadium is more toxic than nickel and at risk for mechanical failure if the surface is scratched, as this element is notch-sensitive. The strength of titanium varies from a value lower than 316L stainless steel to a value equal to the annealed 316L stainless steel. However, when compared by specific strength per density, titanium alloy exceeds other implant material.[2] Titanium has been reported to generate corrosion debris into surrounding soft tissues after implantation as a result of metallic wear. Titanium debris was found in connective tissue, free of macrophage invasion. The debris is a result of the release of titanium dioxide, which is considered to be of low tissue toxicity.[1] To date, the only report of titanium toxicity has been found in dental implants. Surface modifications to titanium have been made in an effort to increase the corrosion resistance of titanium products. Reduction of ion release may extend the implant life and avoid need for removal.

BIOCOMPATIBILITY OF METAL IMPLANTS

The interaction of body tissue and body fluids with the implant is inevitable, and each material will react in its own way, as a form of corrosion with the release of debris into the tissue. The tissue fluid within the human body presents an aggressive environment for corrosion. The effect on the tissue in the body will depend on the type and size of the particles, the concentration and duration of exposure, in addition to the surface characteristics of the implant. Metallic elements can occur in the soft tissue without visible signs of implant corrosion.[5] Metal ions may bind to the body tissue and proteins as soon as they are released from their metallic components. Albumin is abundant in interstitial fluid and serves as an effective transport medium for the ion complexes. The surface-tissue interaction is dynamic and will develop into new stages as time passes.

Corrosion in metals is divided into a variety of interactions.

1. Galvanic corrosion: occurs when 2 dissimilar metals are occurring in the same environment. Galvanic corrosion will occur at the side of the anode, or at the side of the more negative metal. This allows for more rapid corrosion, therefore it is advised that implantation of dissimilar metals is avoided.
2. Fretting corrosion (also known as crevice corrosion): a mechanical rubbing of one part on another, which disrupts the passivation layer, or inert covering, leading to corrosion in an area of low oxygen. This occurs between the contact area of the plate and screw and is most apparent in stainless steel implants.
3. Pitting corrosion: Stainless steel is vulnerable to pitting. Pitting is a form of localized corrosion in which pits form on the metal surface of the plate.

Clinically, corrosion of implants can cause localized pain and irritation, in addition to swelling over the implant. Radiographs may demonstrate subtle metallic particles that are consistent with cracking or flaking of the plate. Surgically, black or gray discoloration can occur within the soft tissues surrounding the implant. Metallosis, which is the release of corrosion debris into the surrounding tissue, can be found on implant removal. Titanium debris is found in the connective tissue, but is free of macrophage invasion, while 316L stainless steel is incorporated into macrophages and giant cell bodies. Titanium dioxide is the ion released from titanium, and is considered low tissue toxicity, compared with the debris from stainless steel.[6]

Titanium implants have minimal corrosion debris due to the passivation layer, which occurs by forming a solid oxide layer. Cobalt-chromium implants are passive as well, and do not exhibit pitting corrosion. The 316L stainless steel is vulnerable to both pitting and crevice corrosion; however, has greater resistance to pitting with the addition of the alloy molybdenum.

The oxide barrier of a stainless steel implant is compromised with bending, scratching, or uneven covering by tissues, which will enhance the corrosion process. Once an implant has been used, it should not be re-used or re-implanted.

The routine removal of metallic implant devices after fracture healing remains an issue of debate. There are no evidence-based guidelines on this matter, despite the documented potential for corrosion of the implant and potential for tissue toxicity. Surgeons representing 65 countries, 571 men and 84 women, completed a survey on implant removal. Of those participants, 58% did not agree that routine implant removal is necessary and 58% did not agree that indwelling implants pose an excess risk for general adverse effects. Forty-eight percent felt that removal is riskier than leaving the implant in place.[7]

CURRENT AVAILABLE IMPLANTS

Metallic implants comprise most implants currently used in foot and ankle surgery. These devices include, but are not limited to wires, pins, staples, screws, plates, implants, joint prosthesis, and 3-dimensional (3D) printed implants.

Wires and Pins

Stainless steel wires and pins are used as guidewires, percutaneous fixation, with the intention that the fixation is temporary, or for permanent fixation of bone not amenable to other fixation. Potential reasons for wire fixation may include osteoporosis, comminution of the fracture fragments, infection, or open injuries with the loss of soft tissue envelope. Most of these devices are manufactured from stainless steel.

Staples

There are several varieties of staples used for osseous fixation, including stainless steel and titanium. They differ in shape, physical properties, and compression capabilities. Biomechanical testing revealed that the stainless steel staple demonstrated the highest fixation stiffness in both bending and torsion, although there was permanent deformation of the staple. The titanium staple provided adequate stiffness, resisted permanent deformation, and was easier to handle.[8]

Screws

There are a plethora of screws available for fixation of the foot and ankle. The earliest screws were made of 316 LVM, and subsequently different alloys of stainless steel have been used with varying success. Screws are offered in many styles, such as solid core, cannulated, cortical, cancellous, fully threaded, partially threaded, headed, and headless. They are made of both stainless steel and titanium; however, titanium has shown to offer an advantage of reduced artifact on advanced imaging after open reduction and internal fixation.[9]

Plates

Plates are frequently used to restore anatomic alignment of the osseous structures within the foot and ankle, and serve to restore functional stability within foot and ankle deformities through osteotomies and arthrodesis procedures. Plates come in a variety of styles, including anatomic, locking, and compression. Plates are constructed of both stainless steel and titanium; however, the trend for titanium constructs is more common given the improved strength under repeated stress, minimal reactivity, and relatively low associated toxicity.

Hammertoe Implant

These implants are designed to fit within the intramedullary canal and span the proximal interphalangeal joint. Some designs promote fixation of the 2 bones, whereas others promote compression of the joint between the 2 bones. They may be made from metals like stainless steel, titanium, and nitinol, or from polyetheretherketone (PEEK), bioabsorbable materials, or human allograft bone. A retrospective review of operative hammertoe correction was performed in 96 patients with a 1-year follow-up. Functional outcome was assessed and no statically significant difference in function outcomes or incidence of complication were observed among the 3 fixation groups. Sixty-five toes (34.9%) were treated with K-wire fixation, 94 (50.5%) with Smart Toe titanium implant, and 27 (14.5%) with TenFuse allograft implant. Implant choice should be based on the patient's need, surgeon experience, and cost of the device.[10]

Metatarsophalangeal Joint Arthroplasty (Total and Hemi)

Total and hemi arthroplasty systems are some of the various implant options available for metatarsophalangeal joint arthroplasty. Hemi, or unipolar, implants initially consisted of silicone and demonstrated a high rate of failure. Design advances and the addition of titanium or cobalt-chromium have improved success of the unipolar implant. The 2-component system, or bipolar implant, have incorporated metallic alloys into the overall implant design. Cobalt-chrome alloys have been used within the metatarsal component and titanium alloys are used in the phalangeal component. The design uses an interface with ultrahigh molecular weight polyethylene to titanium alloys at the phalangeal base. Hemi implants demonstrate greater success due to limited bone resection and preservation of the attachment of the flexor tendon to the base of the phalanx.

Three-Dimensional Printed Implants

The advancement of 3D printing technologies has allowed for the use of custom-designed implants for difficult to treat foot and ankle pathology. Titanium allows for the benefit of unlimited geometry, increased size options over allograft or autograft, and no donor-site morbidity. Titanium alloy implants have mechanical properties similar to those of native bone.[11]

Pyrolytic carbon
This material has been used in the development of joint prosthesis due to its excellent biomechanical properties. It is formed by the pyrolysis of a hydrocarbon gas and has the physical and mechanical properties between graphite and diamond.[12,13] This material has a similar elastic modulus to cortical bone with a higher durability and wear resistance. This minimizes the amount of stress at the bone-implant interface as well as debris and inflammatory reaction. One initial drawback is poor fixation to bone. Biologic fixation of pyrolytic carbon implants can be enhanced by surface texturing with direct exposure to atomic oxygen, without compromising its biocompatibility. Literature is lacking in the application of this prosthesis in human subjects.[14,15]

Thermoplastics
Polyethylene Polyethylene is formed by the polymerization of ethylene. It is currently used as a component of joint arthroplasty. It has minimal, if any, toxicity, and

degradation is a slow process. Polyethylene cannot be sterilized in an autoclave, as this causes permanent degradation of the material. The production of particulate polyethylene debris plays a role in component loosening. The particulate matter forms an inflammatory reaction and causes subsequent bone resorption.[16] Polyethylene is used in ankle implants for total ankle arthroplasty. Highly cross-linked polyethylene has a significantly lower wear rate and produced fewer particles than conventional ultrahigh molecular weight polyethylene. Therefore, highly cross-linked polyethylene could be beneficial in decreasing osteolysis and component loosening in total ankle arthroplasty implants.[17]

Polyetheretherketone PEEK is a thermoplastic known to be a polyketone. It is a semicrystalline thermoplastic that has very strong mechanical properties. Implantable PEEK can be adapted to various stress applications, and can be formulated to match the elasticity of bone. It is resistant to hydrolysis and ionizing radiation, and therefore, it is unaffected by conventional sterilization techniques. It can be found in subtalar arthroereisis implants, interphalangeal joint implants, and bone anchors for the foot and ankle.[2]

Bioceramics

This term encompasses the use of ceramic materials to augment or replace various parts of the body. Compounds include silicates, metallic oxides, carbides, refractory hybrids, sulfides, and selenides. Material must be nontoxic, noncarcinogenic, nonallergic, noninflammatory, and biocompatible to be classified as a bioceramic. It is important for the bioceramic to have the density and strength to mimic the surrounding bone, and should not be significantly stronger to reduce the risk of stress shielding.

Bioceramics have poor mechanical properties, being brittle and unable to withstand compressive loads.[18] The structural characteristics of bioceramics can be improved with hot pressing or sintering, as exposure to high pressure and temperature will produce a more uniform crystalline structure with improved ability to manage load-bearing forces.

There are nonabsorbable and absorbable bioceramics available. Nonabsorbable ceramics are used to make implants and use aluminum oxide.[19] Small grain and higher porosity of the aluminum oxide will yield a stronger implant. The advantage of this material is excellent wear resistance, stability, and inertness. Biodegradable (or absorbable) ceramics include aluminum calcium phosphate, coralline, plaster of Paris, hydroxyapatite (HA), and tricalcium phosphate. They are mainly used for resorbable bone substitutes for filling bone defects and usage in drug delivery systems. Calcium phosphate when used in graft form is an excellent option for filling defects that do not require stability, as the high concentrations of calcium and phosphate activate osteoblasts to produce bone.[20] Calcium sulfate is used as a bone graft substitute; however, does not provide osteoconductive properties due to the rapidly dissolving properties of this material. This is best used in filling bone defects from trauma or deficits following evacuation of cysts.[21] Calcium phosphate and calcium sulfate can be combined as graft material. Animal studies show the combination of the 2 bioceramics demonstrates greater compressive strength compared with pure calcium sulfate and normal bone at 13 and 26 weeks after implantation[22] with an elastic modulus comparable to restored bone. Current indications are similar to other ceramics and used for void filler in bony deficits related to trauma.

Hydroxyapatite HA is converted from coral through a hydrothermal exchange process and is an osteoconductive material. It is used to fill defects, as it cannot withstand physiologic loads on initial implantation. The integration process involves fibrovascular ingrowth with osteoblasts, producing new bone on the porous surface of the hydroxyapatite. Once the graft is incorporated by the host bone, it can then withstand loads.

Polymethylmethacrylate Polymethylmethacrylate (PMMA) is a composite biomaterial that is space-filling and load transferring. It will not bond chemically to bone or metallic surfaces; however, if the implant surface is textured, bonding can occur in an operating room setting. PMMA is brittle once hardened, and can withstand substantial compressive force. PMMA can be mixed with a powder form of antibiotics, and serves as a delivery system. Heat-stable antibiotics are a requirement, as polymerization of PMMA is an exothermic process. Three factors will cause PMMA to elicit a reaction of local tissues:

1. Heat polymerization that exceeds the coagulation temperature of proteins
2. Occlusion of nutrient metaphyseal articles resulting in bone necrosis
3. Cytotoxic and lipolytic reaction of the nonpolymerized monomer

Histologically, these tissues are damaged within the initial 21 days following surgery, and the repair process can last for up to 2 years.[23]

SUMMARY

There are a variety of materials available for surgical reconstruction of the foot and ankle. When considering the type of material, the application of the material should be taken into consideration, and one that provides the best physical properties to match the mechanical stress should be chosen. With metallic implants, the potential for corrosion and tissue reactivity should be taken into consideration, as both stainless steel and titanium alloys are comparable in strength. With the advancements in the application of titanium alloys, custom-designed implants provide an alternative option for patients with complex foot and ankle pathology or trauma. It is to be hoped that further developments in metallurgy will allow the development of new alloys that, when compared with current alloys, will have better mechanical and physical properties yielding better long-term results with implants.

With the expanding magnitude and diversity of implant materials, including ceramics and modified polyethylenes, there will be improvement in the longevity of total joint replacements with alternative bearing surfaces and with the addition of composite materials.

Material for the fabrication of the ideal implant is still unknown; however, a more biocompatible material is desired to produce less antigenicity and reactivity. The least reactive materials should be considered for implantation that still provide appropriate physical properties to withstand the stress and strain of the surrounding tissues in order to optimize patient outcomes and satisfaction.

REFERENCES

1. Chang TJ, Werd MB, Hovelsen C. Metallic implants used in foot surgery. Clin Podiatr Med Surg 1995;12:457–74.
2. Grambart ST, Christensen JT. Biomaterials: metals and other nonabsorbables. In: Southerland JT, editor. McGlamry's comprehensive textbook of foot and ankle surgery. 4th edition. Philadelphia: Wolters Kluwer Health|Lippincott Williams & Wilkins; 2013. p. 15–23.
3. Ferguson AB, Laing PG, Hodge ES. The ionization of metal implants in living tissues. J Bone Joint Surg Am 1960;42:77.

4. Heath JC, Freeman MA, Swanson SA. Carcinogenic properties of wear particles from prostheses made in cobalt-chromium alloy. Lancet 1971;1(7699):564–6.

5. Scales JT, Winter GT, Shirley HT. Corrosion of orthopedic implants. J Bone Joint Surg Br 1959;41:810–20.

6. Rosenberg A, Gratz KW, Sailer HF. Should titanium miniplates be removed after bone healing is complete? Int J Oral Maxillofac Surg 1993;22(3):185–8.

7. Hanson B, Van Der Werken C, Stengel D. Surgeons' beliefs and perceptions about removal of orthopaedic implants. BMC Musculoskelet Disord 2008;9:73.

8. Rethnam U, Kuiper J, Makwana N. Mechanical characteristics of three staples commonly used in foot surgery. J Foot Ankle Res 2009;2:5.

9. Radzi S, Cowin G, Robinson M, et al. Metal artifacts from titanium and steels screws in CT, 1.5T and 3T MR images of the tibial pilon: a quantitative assessment in 3D. Quant Imaging Med Surg 2014;4:163–72.

10. Obrador C, Losa-Iglesias M, Bercerro-de-Bengoa-Vallego R, et al. Comparative study of intramedullary hammertoe fixation. Foot Ankle Int 2018;39:415–25.

11. Dekker TJ, Steele JR, Federer AE, et al. Use of patient-specific 3D-printed titanium implants for complex foot and ankle limb salvage, deformity correction, and arthrodesis procedures. Foot Ankle Int 2018;39(8):916–21.

12. Parker WL, Rizzo M, Moran SL, et al. Preliminary results of nonconstrained pyrolytic carbon arthroplasty for metacarpophalangeal joint arthritis. J Hand Surg Am 2007;32(10):1496–505.

13. Haubold AD. On the durability of pyrolytic carbon in vivo. Med Prog Technol 1994;20(3–4):201–18.

14. Hetherington VJ, Kawalec JS, Bhattacharyya B. Enhancement of the fixation of pyrolytic carbon implants by using atomic oxygen texturing. J Foot Ankle Surg 2004;43(1):16–9.

15. Apard T, Casin C, Moubarak E, et al. A novel pyrolytic carbon implant for hallux rigidus: a cadaveric study. J Foot Ankle Surg 2011;17(3):182–5.

16. Kurtz SM, Jewett CW, Foulds JR, et al. A miniature specimen mechanical testing technique scaled to articulating surface of polyethylene components for total joint arthroplasty. J Biomed Mater Res 1999;48(1):75–81.

17. Schipper ON, Haddad SL, Fullam S, et al. Wear characteristics of conventional ultrahigh-molecular-weight polyethylene versus highly cross-linked polyethylene in total ankle arthroplasty. Foot Ankle Int 2018;39(11):1335–44.

18. Szabo G, Schmidt B. Mechanical properties of bone after grafting with coralline hydroxyapatite: an experimental study. Orthopedics 1993;16(2):197–8.

19. Rush SM. Bone graft substitutes: osteobiologics. Clin Podiatr Med Surg 2005; 22(4):619–30, viii.

20. Elsner A, Jubel A, Prokop A, et al. Augmentation of intraarticular calcaneal fractures with injectable calcium phosphate cement: densitometry, histology, and functional outcome of 18 patients. J Foot Ankle Surg 2005;44(5):390–5.

21. Thordarson DB, Bollinger M. SRS cancellous bone cement augmentation of calcaneal fracture fixation. Foot Ankle Int 2005;26(5):347–52.

22. Urban RM, Turner TM, Hall DJ, et al. Increased bone formation using calcium sulfate-calcium phosphate composite graft. Clin Orthop Relat Res 2007;459: 110–7.

23. Lidgren L, Drar H, Moller J. Strength of polymethylmethacrylate increased by vacuum mixing. Acta Orthop Scand 1984;55(5):536–41.

Updates in Tendinopathy Treatment Options

Meagan M. Jennings, DPM[a],*, Victoria Liew, BS[b], Breana Marine, BS[b]

KEYWORDS

- Achilles tendinopathy • Tendinopathy • Tendonitis

KEY POINTS

- Advances made in the understanding of the tendinopathy disease process includes inflammation as part of the early tendinopathy process.
- Once thought to not contribute to the early process of tendon degeneration, this hypothesis has now been refuted. This allows some guidance in conservative treatment of the disease process.
- However, when the standard conservative treatments fail, there are some minimally invasive injections such as cell therapy and platelet-rich plasma, as well as ultrasonic debridement techniques, that offer an intermediate treatment step to patients with low-reported morbidity.

TENDINOPATHY PATHOGENESIS

Tendinopathy is a common but disabling condition for many people. It is a term used to describe a complex, multifaceted pathology of the tendon characterized by pain, decreased function, and reduced exercise tolerance.[1,2] This disease process poses an important clinical problem and accounts for up to 30% of general practice musculoskeletal consultations.[3] Researchers still have varying hypotheses as to the underlying pathogenesis of tendinopathy and the efficacy of anti-inflammatory mediators and immunocytes in this disease process. Understanding the mechanisms of inflammation and existing anti-inflammatory and regenerative therapies is key to the development of therapeutic strategies in tendinopathy.

Degeneration or Inflammation?

Initially, the onset of tendinopathy is caused by many factors, particularly physical overuse. In response to this overuse, noninflammatory reactions arise in the tendon

No Disclosures.

[a] Silicon Valley Foot and Ankle Reconstructive Surgery Fellowship, Palo Alto Medical Foundation, 701 E. El Camino Real South Wing, Mountain View, CA 94040, USA; [b] California College of Podiatric Medicine, Samuel Merritt University, 3100 Telegraph Ave, Oakland, CA 94609, USA
* Corresponding author.
E-mail address: mmjfootankle@gmail.com

including thickening and increasing firmness of the tendon.[4] If physical overuse persists, this will ultimately lead to tendon self-repair failure, and the tendon tissue will become disordered and lead to degenerative tendinopathy.[5] Tendon specimens from symptomatic patients exhibit degenerative changes such as being hypoxic, mucoid, hyaline, myxoid, and showing fatty degeneration[6] as well as demonstrate changes to the paratenon.[7]

In the 1970s, Puddu and colleagues[8] found that acute inflammatory cells do not play a role in chronic tendinopathy. It was thought that inflammation had no role in tendinopathy, but some more recent studies have found evidence of early inflammatory responses in tendinopathy.[9,10] With the advancement of immunohistochemistry and molecular biology techniques, the concept of degenerative tendon disease has become less convincing.[11] It is hypothesized that there is a continuous transition from physiologic to pathologic processes in tendon. With this theory, it is assumed that microdamages to tendon fibers occur, and the body then secretes various substances to promote healing, including inflammatory factors.[12]

In the pathogenesis of tendinopathy, inflammation and degeneration may not be 2 separate processes as there appears to be interaction of the 2 processes. A degenerative process may be triggered by inflammation, and inflammation will play some role in later degenerative processes too.[13] Thus, it is safe to say that in the early phases of tendinopathy, people need to use some anti-inflammatory medications to inhibit the progression of this disease. During the late stages of the disease, inflammation has subsided, which means that anti-inflammatory treatments have no value. Because of the poor regenerative capacity of tendon, patients may need to use regenerative medicine strategies to promote healing of tendon.

Inflammation plays an important role in the development of tendinopathy, and there are numerous inflammatory mediators in this continuum of degeneration that may be areas of targeted therapy in the future; however, the individual mediators will not be elaborated upon in this text. To a certain extent, anti-inflammatory therapy can effectively inhibit the progress of tendon diseases in the early stages. However, there is little inflammation in the later stages of tendon disease and torn tendon. Thus, other strategies for tendon repair are needed for the noninflammatory disease state of tendons such as tissue engineering-based therapy.

The thought that tendinopathy may be purely an inflammatory disease is incomplete. Other contributing factors to tendinopathy include compression with pulling force on the tendon. Although low mechanical stimulation can upregulate the expression of tenocyte-related genes in tendon stem cells, mechanical overloading can lead to increased expression of both tenocyte-related and nontenocyte-related genes.[14] And while overuse is one of the main causative factors of tendinopathy, there appears to be a complex relationship between inflammation, mechanics, and degenerative changes. Thus, more studies are needed exploring this dynamic process.

Achilles Insertional Tendinopathy

Pulling force on a tendon can be termed overuse and can cause tendinopathy; however, pulling force in eccentric exercise can also treat tendinopathy. During physical activities, there are compression and pulling forces. There are 2 types of compression during tendon activity. One is a direct contact on the tendon, and the other type of compression exists at the bone-tendon interface. In Achilles insertional tendinopathy, pathology associated with a Haglund deformity (direct compression), is caused by the bone pushing on the tendon while there is a pulling force. The second type of Achilles insertional tendinopathy is with another type of indirect compression and is dependent upon the direction of tendon force. If the tendon force is perpendicular to the bone surface (the tendon pulls straight vertical), there will be no compression; however, if the tendon is subjected to angular tension, the side of the tendon nearest bone will be under compression and can present as enthesopathy and eventually, Achilles insertional calcific tendinosis (AICT). Combinations of these 2 load types most likely induce tissue pathology.[15]

The term impingement refers to a form of mechanical load that adds compressive or shearing load to the normal tensile load on the tendon. Bullock and colleagues[16] showed with MRI that there is more Achilles tendinopathy in close proximity to the superior aspect of the calcaneal tuberosity, which is consistent with impingement in 67.5% of subjects. They suggested that Achilles impingement tendinopathy would be a more appropriate terminology for Haglund syndrome, as Haglund syndrome refers to the impingement (or direct compression) of the retrocalcaneal bursa and Achilles tendon.

Theoretically, then, one can assume that a Haglund deformity syndrome is caused by direct compression on the side of the tendon that is near the bone. Axial loading of the tendon (overuse) plus compression on the tendon causes pathology of the tendon side nearest the bone, while the posterior side will remain normal. As for AICT, compression and pulling force can initially provoke paratenon inflammation. The upregulation of inflammatory mediators and immunocytes can lead to increasing numbers of abnormal phenotype tenoncytes and cause proliferation of peripheral blood vessels and the onset of calcification.[15] Both of these conditions hypothetically cause the first inflammatory phase and peritendinitis, which subsequently, will exert an adverse effect on the tendon itself. Puddu and colleagues[8] proposed a classification system of Achilles tendon disease, which included pure peritendinitis, peritendinitis with tendinosis, and tendinosis. In some cases of peritendinitis, they found marked vascular proliferation in the peritendon that tended to invade the normal tendon. Mesenchymal cell types then can invade the tendon tissue in a disorganized fashion and cause irregularly oriented collagen.[8] Thus, one can conclude all degenerative tendon pathology starts with an the peritendon inflammatory process.

Achilles Midsubstance Tendinopathy

The underlying etiology for Achilles midsubstance tendinopathy has many theories without a specific, clear understanding. Everything from tendon vascularity, tendon dysfunction, age, sex, body weight and height, pes cavus, and lateral ankle instability can be common intrinsic factors. Excessive motion of the hindfoot in the frontal plane, especially a lateral heel strike with excessive compensatory protonation, is thought to cause a whipping action on the Achilles tendon and predispose it to tendinopathy.[6] Changes in training patterns, poor techniques, previous injuries, footwear, and environmental factors such as training on hard or slanting surfaces are extrinsic factors that may predispose the athlete to Achilles tendinopathy. Excessive loading of tendons during vigorous physical training is regarded as the main pathologic stimulus for tendinopathy,[17] possibly as a result of imbalance between muscle power and tendon elasticity. The Achilles may respond to repetitive overload by either inflammation of its sheath, degeneration of its body, or a combination of both.[18,19] It may still be important to discern paratendon lesions from tendon lesions. The painful arc sign differentiates this on clinical examination. In paratendinopathy, the area of maximum thickening and tenderness remains fixed in relation to the malleoli from full dorsiflexion to plantarflexion, whereas lesions within the tendon move with ankle motion. There is often a discrete tendon nodule whose tenderness significantly decreases or disappears when the tendon is put under tension.[20]

Degenerative tendinopathy is the most common histologic finding in spontaneous tendon ruptures. Tendon degeneration may lead to reduced tensile strength and a predisposition to rupture. In Achilles tendinopathy, changes in the expression of genes regulating cell-to-cell and cell-to-matrix interactions have been reported with down-regulation of MMP3 and mRNA.[21] Significantly higher levels of type I and type III collagen mRNAs have been reported in tendinopathic samples compared with normal samples. Thus, tendinopathy and its associated pain must include a combination of mechanical and biochemical causes.[22]

CONSERVATIVE TENDINOPATHY MANAGEMENT

Despite the morbidity associated with Achilles tendinopathy, management is still not 100% scientifically based. Managements that have been investigated with random-ized controlled trials include nonsteroidal anti-inflammatory drugs (NSAIDs),[23,24] eccentric exercise,[25–32] glyceryl trinitrate patches,[33–35] sclerosing injections,[36,37] and shock wave treatment.[38]

It is thought that surgery should be reserved until patients have failed conservative therapy for at least 6 months. Despite the abundance of therapeutic options, few ran-domized prospective, placebo, controlled trials exist to assist in choosing the best management.[39]

Acute tendinopathy is actually a well-advanced failure of a chronic healing response in which there is neither histologic nor biochemical evidence of inflammation.[6] Howev-er, as described previously, newer literature supports the upregulation in inflammatory mediators in the earliest phases of tendinopathy, and in fact the acute phase of ten-dinopathy, some would suggest should technically be termed paratendonitis, as evi-dence suggests inflammatory mediators are upregulated.[15] Thus, within the first few weeks of symptom onset, treatment with anti-inflammatory drugs should be started even though this has been reported as controversial.[6] Oral NSAIDs used for a short term can provide symptomatic relief. Oral NSAID therapy daily, cryotherapy multiple times daily, protection of the tendon via immobilization (cast boot) or off-loading (heel lifts), avoidance of incline/decline and dynamic training should be implemented. Further stretching on the tendon during this acute phase typically will induce more in-flammatory cells, so this should be avoided during the acute phase of treatment. Acute phase treatment shall be implemented for 7 to 10 days until acute inflammatory type symptoms resolve. Some tenderness may still be present and certainly tendon thick-ening if present, will not have resolved.

After the initial acute inflammatory phase of a paratendonitis/early stage tendinop-athy has subsided, therapeutic treatment focusing on tendon strengthening and reor-ganization of collagen should occur. Typically, this involves an eccentric training program which has been referenced in various numerous studies and studied in ran-domized controlled trials.[25–32] Some discomfort is usually still present during this phase and additional therapeutic modalities by a physical therapist should be pre-scribed. Decreasing everyday load demands on the tendon are still appropriate via heel lifts, orthotic support or even immobilization while the patient continues to work on tendon strengthening and flexibility.

When treatment through the first phases of the tendinopathy process has not been successful for a minimum of 6 months, other modalities may be considered. Depending on the impact of the patient's symptoms on quality of life, one may consider invasive treatment modalities at this time. Advanced imaging may also be indicated at this stage to further assess the amount of tendon degeneration and involvement.

INVASIVE TENDINOPATHY TREATMENT

Regenerative medicine has the ultimate aim of finding effective ways to promote self-repair and regeneration and restore the injured tissue to normal function. In the treatment of tendinopathy, there are several different strategies to promote tendon regeneration: growth factors, cells, biomaterials, and mechanical debridement.

Growth Factors

During the early repair process following tendon injury, upregulating the expression of some growth factors is beneficial for tendon healing.[40,41] These factors include: basic fibroblast growth factor (bFGF), insulin-like growth factor (IGF-1), Platelet-derived growth factor (PDGF), transforming growth factor-β (TGFβT), and vascular endothelial growth factor (VEGF); all play diverse roles during the healing process.[41–43] The synergy of these factors has a more productive effect.

Platelet-Rich Plasma

The use of platelet-rich plasma (PRP) is controversial, and preparation methods may complicate interpretation of efficacy. More studies are now available on PRP; however, there is no clear consensus on the efficacy in Achilles tendinopathy. Zhou and colleagues[44] stated that PRP can promote tenocyte proliferation in vitro, and accelerate proliferation rates of circulating stem cells, ultimately contributing to overall tendon healing. Although PRP can induce tendon stem cells to differentiate into tenocytes, it cannot reverse nontenocyte differentiation. PRP can increase the total collagen synthesis in both tenocytes and tendon stem cells, and enhances gene expression of collagen types 1 and 3, which allows growth and healing to injured tendons.

Gosens and colleagues[45] performed a high-quality, randomized controlled trial that demonstrated that autologous PRP injections have better cure rates and pain scores than cortisone injections for up to 2 years after treatment in lateral epicondylitis. Jo and colleagues[46] looked at the effects of PRP with concomitant use of a corticosteroid on tenocytes and found that the addition of PRP did not influence the anti-inflammatory effects of the corticosteroid, but it ameliorated the deleterious adverse effects of the corticosteroid.

The variability of PRP components makes its use in clinical therapy somewhat unpredictable and controversial. Yan and colleagues[47] studied the influence of leukocytes on PRP-mediated tissue healing. They found that leucocyte-poor PRP improved tendon healing with better histologic results in a rabbit Achilles model, which may be a better option for clinical treatment of tendinopathy compared with leucocyte-rich PRP.

Thus, leukocyte-poor PRP can be considered a low-morbidity treatment for Achilles tendinopathy. It offers patients an in-office treatment modality that has shown great promise in promoting tendon repair and symptomatic relief.

STEM CELLS

In regenerative medicine, stem cell therapy can exert beneficial effects on the musculoskeletal system and encompasses a broad range of cell types such as bone mesenchymal stem cells (BMSCs), tendon stem/progenitor cells (TSPCs), adipose -derived mesenchymal stem cells (ADMSCs), and embryonic stem cells (ESCs). All of these cell types can exert a positive effect on tendon healing. Studies have shown that in rotator cuff repair with BMSC injections, there were a reported reduced number of ruptures over time.[48,49] ADMSCs were shown in a pilot study to significantly improve lateral epicondylitis.[50] To date, there have not been any published clinical studies to describe the therapeutic effects of TSPCs and ESCs; however, there is evidence to support and validate the self-renewal and differentiation capacity of these cell types. More high-level clinical trials are necessary to validate the efficacy and safety of cell therapy.

BIOMATERIALS

Engineered tendon tissue is possible with newer technologies. Tendon scaffold materials can provide support and protection for cells, but more importantly, the interaction of cells with scaffold materials can affect cell survival, migration, proliferation, and metabolism. Natural biomaterials include collagen silk, hyaluronic acid, alginate, and decellularized tendon xenografts.[51] A woven silk-collagen sponge scaffold similar to natural tendon with superior mechanical characteristics has been developed.[52] A bioactive knitted silk-collagen sponge scaffold that can release stromal cell-derived factor 1α (SDF-1α) and thus enhance the number of local fibroblast-like cells and inhibit the accumulation of immunocytes, which enhanced repair of injured tendon, also has been developed.[53] Biomaterials may unlock some wonderful advances in the field of tendon tissue repair.

MECHANICAL DEBRIDEMENT

Ultrasonic debridement is a technology that has shown promise in other areas of medicine. Studies have shown success via percutaneous treatments by ultrasonic debridement. A minimally invasive procedure using ultrasound imaging guidance, Ultrasonic debridement can selectively remove damaged tendon tissue. This induces an acute injury to the tendon as well as removes diseased tissue to stimulate tendon healing and hopefully alleviate pain. Kamineni and colleagues[54] injected collagenase into white rabbits to promote collagen breakdown associated with tendinopathy. Three weeks after manual injection of collagenase, the rabbits were treated with a Tenex ultrasonic probe under ultrasound-visualized guidance, and euthanized 3 weeks later. Tendons were then harvested, treated, and analyzed. The tendons showed more mature and immature fibroblast, less mononuclear cell infiltration, and an aligned pattern of collagen fibers with tissue regeneration. Neovascularization was also present. Major effects of ultrasonic treatment provided regrowth, and the tendon returned to the normal state.

TENDON AUGMENTATION

Tendon transfer to assist in the alleviation of tendinopathy is often saved as the final surgical treatment approach in tendinopathy. Achilles tendinopathy will be focused on in this article.

The flexor hallucis longus (FHL) tendon transfer for tendinopathy of the Achilles tendon has grown more popular among surgical treatments in recent years. Howell and colleagues[55] reported on the use of the FHL tendon to treat AICT after giving unsuccessful conservative treatment for 3 to 6 months. Forty-five patients were included in the study, and 33 patients returned for follow-up. Of the 33 patients who returned, none had a need for revision surgery. The patients also self-reported satisfaction, and 84.8% said they were "very satisfied" with their outcome. The authors concluded that the FHL tendon transfer for AICT is an effective intervention and that more prospective measures should be taken to verify the advantages of the treatment.

Typically, during this procedure, the FHL tendon can be harvested through the same incision used to approach the Achilles tendon off the posteromedial border of the Achilles. FHL harvest through the single posterior incision offers enough tendon to perform the transfer versus needing to harvest it distally near the medial arch. Mao and colleagues[56] reported from 64 specimens that medial and lateral nerve injuries did not occur any more frequently after performing a single minimally invasive incision to harvest the FHL tendon compared with double and single incision techniques. The study did conclude that harvesting the tendon at Henry knot is not recommended because of its close proximity to the medial plantar nerve.

After harvest of the FHL tendon, the senior author's recommendation is to anchor the tendon to the calcaneus via a bone-tendon anchor and perform a tenodesis with the Achilles tendon. This technique offers a failsafe mechanism if 1 attachment mechanism or the other were to fail. There are various anchoring and tensioning techniques for this tendon transfer, which can be referenced in foot and ankle surgery textbooks.

SUMMARY

In summary, understanding of Achilles tendinopathy and tendinopathy in general is still not complete. Advances made in the understanding of the tendinopathy disease process now include inflammation as part of the early tendinopathy process. Once thought to not contribute to the early process of tendon degeneration, this hypothesis has now been refuted. This allows some guidance in conservative treatment of the disease process. However, when the standard conservative treatments fail, there are some minimally invasive injections such as cell therapy and PRP, as well as ultrasonic debridement techniques that offer an intermediate treatment step to patients with low reported morbidity. Certainly, surgical intervention with or without tendon transfer and augmentation is still reserved for those patients in whom no other treatment has been successful.

REFERENCES

1. Riley G. Chronic tendon pathology: molecular basis and therapeutic implications. Expert Rev Mol Med 2005;7:1–25.
2. Andres BM, Murrell GA. Treatment of tendinopathy: what works, what does not, and what is on the horizon. Clin Orthop Relat Res 2008;466:1539–54.
3. McGonagle D, Marzo-Ortega H, Benjamin M, et al. Report on the second international enthesitis workshop. Arthritis Rheum 2003;48:896–905.
4. Aspland CA, Best TM. Achilles tendon disorders. BMJ 2013;346:f1262.
5. Cook JL, Purdam CR. Is tendon pathology a continuum? A pathology model to explain the clinical presentation of load-induced tendinopathy. Br J Sports Med 2009;43:409–16.
6. Longo UG, Ronga M, Maffulli N. Achilles tendinopathy. Sports Med Arthrosc Rev 2018;26:16–30.
7. Maffulli N, Sharma P, Luscombe KL. Achilles tendinopathy: aetiology and management. J R Soc Med 2004;97:472–6.
8. Puddu G, Ippolito E, Postacchini F. A classification of Achilles tendon disease. Am J Sports Med 1976;4:145–50.
9. Millar NL, Murrell GA, McInnes IB. Inflammatory mechanisms in tendinopathy – towards translation. Nat Rev Rheumatol 2017;13:110–22.
10. Millar NL, Hueber AJ, Reilly JH, et al. Inflammation is present in early human tendinopathy. Am J Sports Med 2010;38:2085–91.
11. Rees JD, Stride M, Scott A. Tendons – time to revisit inflammation. Br J Sports Med 2014;48:1553–7.

12. Abate M, Silbernagel KG, Siljeholm C, et al. Pathogenesis of tendinopathies: inflammation or degeneration. Arthritis Res Ther 2009;11:235.
13. Speed C. Inflammation in tendon disorders. Adv Exp Med Biol 2016;920:209–20.
14. Zhang J, Wang JH. The effects of mechanical loading on tendons – an in vivo and in vitro model study. PLoS One 2013;8:e71740.
15. Tang C, Chen Y, Huang J, et al. The roles of inflammatory mediators and immunocytes in tendinopathy. J Orthop Translat 2018;14:23–33.
16. Bullock MJ, Mourelatos J, Mar A. Achilles impingement tendinopathy on magnetic resonance imaging. J Foot Ankle Surg 2017;56:555–63.
17. Leadbetter WB. Cell-matrix response in tendon injury. Clin Sports Med 1992;11: 533–78.
18. Johnson KW, Zalavras C, Thordarson DB. Surgical management of insertional calcific Achilles tendinosis with a central tendon splitting approach. Foot Ankle Int 2006;27:245–50.
19. Kvist M. Achilles tendon injuries in athletes. Sports Med 1994;18:173–201.
20. Barnes SJ, Gey van Pettius D, Maffulli N. Angioleiomyoma of the Achilles tendon. Bull Hosp Jt Dis 2003;61:137–9.
21. Sharma P, Maffulli N. Understanding and managing Achilles tendinopathy. Br J Hosp Med (Lond) 2006;67:64–7.
22. Maffulli N, Benazzo F. Basic sciences of tendons. Sports Med Arthrosc Rev 2000; 8:1–5.
23. Forsland C, Bylander B, Aspenberg P. Indomethacin and celecoxib improve tendon healing in rats. Acta Orthop Scand 2003;74:465–9.
24. Virchenko O, Skoglund B, Aspenberg P. Parecoxib impairs early tendon repair but improves later remodeling. Am J Sports Med 2004;32:1–5.
25. Mafi N, Lorentzon R, Alfredson H. Superior short-term concentric training in a randomized prospective multicenter study on patients with chronic Achilles tendinosis. Knee Surg Sports Traumatol Arthrosc 2001;9:42–7.
26. Alfredson H, Pietila T, Jonsson P, et al. Heavy-load eccentric calf muscle training for treatment of chronic Achilles tendinosis. Am J Sports Med 1998;26:360–6.
27. Sayana Mk, Maffulli N. Eccentric calf muscle training in non-athletic patients with Achilles tendinopathy. J Sci Med Sport 2007;10:52–8.
28. Rompe JD, Nafe B, Furia JP, et al. Eccentric loading, shock-wave treatment, or a wait-and-see policy for tendinopathy of the main body of the tendo Achilles: a randomized controlled trial. Am J Sports Med 2007;35:374–83.
29. Maffulli N, Longo UG. How do eccentric exercises work in tendinopathy? Rheumatology 2008;47:1444–5.
30. Rompe JD, Furia JP, Maffulli N. Eccentric loading versus eccentric loading plus shock wave treatment for mid-portion Achilles tendinopathy: a randomized controlled trial. Am J Sports Med 2009;37:463–70.
31. Knobloch K, Schreibmueller L, Longo UG, et al. Eccentric exercises for the management of tendinopathy of the main body of the Achilles tendon with or without an AirHeeltrade mark Brace. A randomized controlled trial. B: effects of compliance. Disabil Rehabil 2008;30:1692–6.
32. Knobloch K, Schreibmueller L, Longo UG, et al. Eccentric exercises for the management of tendinopathy of the main body of the Achilles tendon with or without an AirHeeltrade mark Brace. A randomized controlled trial. A: effects on pain and microcirculation. Disabil Rehabil 2008;30:1685–91.
33. Paoloni JA, Murrell GA. Three-year follow-up study of topical glyceryl trinitrate treatment of chronic noninsertional Achilles tendinopathy. Foot Ankle Int 2007; 28:1064–8.

34. Paoloni JA, Appleyard RC, Nelson J, et al. Topical glyceryl trinitrate and noninsertional Achilles tendinopathy. A randomized, double-blind, placebo-controlled trial. J Bone Joint Surg Am 2004;86-A:916–22.

35. Kane TP, Ismail M, Calder JD. Topical glyceryl trinitrate and noninsertional Achilles tendinopathy: a clinical and cellular investigation. Am J Sports Med 2008;36:1160–3.

36. Hoksrud A, Ohberg L, Alfredson H, et al. Ultrasound-guided sclerosis of neovessels in painful chronic patellar tendinopathy: a randomized controlled trial. Am J Sports Med 2006;34:1738–46.

37. Maxwell NJ, Ryan MD, Taunton JE, et al. Sonographically guided intratendinous injection of hyperosmolar dextrose to treat chronic tendinosis of the Achilles tendon: a pilot study. Am J Roentgenol 2007;189:W215–20.

38. Giombini A, Giovannini V, Di Cesare A, et al. Hyperthermia induced by microwave diathermy in the management of muscle and tendon injuries. Br Med Bull 2007;83:379–96.

39. Rompe JD, Furia JP, Maffulli N. Mid-portion Achilles tendinopathy – current options for treatment. Disabil Rehabil 2008;30:1666–76.

40. Heisterbach PE, Todorov A, Fluckiger R, et al. Effect of BMP-12, TGF-β1 ad autologous conditioned serum on growth factor expression in Achilles tendon healing. Knee Surg Sports Traumatol Arthrosc 2012;20:1907–14.

41. Wurgler-Hauri CC, Dourte LM, Baradet TC, et al. Temporal expression of 8 growth factors in tendon-to-bone healing in a rat supraspinatus model. J Shoulder Elbow Surg 2007;16:S198–203.

42. Chen CH, Cao Y, Wu YR, et al. Tendon healing in vivo: gene expression and production of multiple growth factors in early tendon period. J Hand Surg Am 2008;33:1834–42.

43. Orchard J, Kountouris A. The management of tennis elbow. BMJ 2011;342:d2687.

44. Zhou Y, Wang J. PRP treatment efficacy for tendinopathy: a review of basic science studies. Biomed Res Int 2016;9103792. https://doi.org/10.1155/2016/9103792.

45. Gosens T, Peerbooms JC, van Laar W, et al. Ongoing positive effect of platelet-rich plasma versus corticosteroid injection in lateral epicondylitis: a double-blind randomized controlled trial with 2-year follow-up. Am J Sports Med 2011;39:1200–8.

46. Jo CH, Lee SY, Yoon KS, et al. Effects of platelet-rich plasma with concomitant use of a corticosteroid on tenocytes from degenerative rotator cuff tears in interleukin 1β-induced tendinopathic conditions. Am J Sports Med 2017;45:1141–50.

47. Yan R, Gu Y, Ran J, et al. Intratendon delivery of leukocyte-poor platelet-rich plasma improves healing compared with leukocyte-rich platelet-rich plasma in a rabbit Achilles tendinopathy model. Am J Sports Med 2017;45:1909–20.

48. Ellera GJL, da SRC, Silla LM, et al. Conventional rotator cuff repair complemented by the aid of mononuclear autologous stem cells. Knee Surg Sports Traumatol Arthrosc 2012;20:373–7.

49. Hernigou P, Flouzat LCH, Delambre J, et al. Biologic augmentation of rotator cuff repair with mesenchymal stem cells during arthroscopy improves healing and prevents further tears: a case-controlled study. Int Orthop 2014;38:1811–8.

50. Lee SY, Kim W, Lim C, et al. Treatment of lateral epicondylosis by using allogeneic adipose-derived mesenchymal stem cells: a pilot study. Stem Cells 2015;33:2995–3005.

51. Docheva D, Muller SA, Majewski M, et al. Biologics for tendon repair. Adv Drug Deliv Rev 2015;84:222–39.
52. Zheng Z, Ran J, Chen W, et al. Alignment of collagen fiber in knitted silk scaffold for functional massive rotator cuff repair. Acta Biomater 2017;51:317–29.
53. Shen W, Chen X, Chen J, et al. The effect of incorporation of exogenous stromal cell-derived factor 1-alpha within a knitted silk-collagen sponge scaffold on tendon regeneration. Biomaterials 2010;31:7239–49.
54. Kamineni S, Butterfield T, Sinai A, et al. "Percutaneous ultrasonic debridement of tendinopathy—a pilot achilles rabbit model. J Orthop Surg Res 2015;10:70.
55. Howell MA, McConn TP, Saltrick KR, et al. Calcific insertional Achilles tendinopathy-Achilles repair with flexor hallucis longus tendon transfer: case series and surgical technique. J Foot Ankle Surg 2019;58(2):236–42.
56. Mao H, Dong W, Shi Z, et al. Anatomical study of the neurovascular in flexor hallucis longus tendon transfers. Sci Rep 2017;7(1):14202.

Flexible Fixation in Foot and Ankle Surgery

Katherine M. Raspovic, DPM*, Kendall Anigian, MD, Jaclyn Kapilow, MD, Breann Tisano, MD

KEYWORDS

- Flexible fixation • Suture-button • Suture-tape • Syndesmosis repair
- Lisfranc disruption • Spring ligament augmentation
- Lateral ankle ligament augmentation

KEY POINTS

- Flexible fixation devices have been described and used for syndesmotic injuries and augmentation of lateral ankle ligament repair.
- Flexible fixation devices have been described and used in cases of Lisfranc ligamentous disruption, hallux valgus, hallux varus repair, and more recently spring ligament repair augmentation.
- Use of these devices continues to evolve in foot and ankle surgery.

INTRODUCTION

Flexible fixation has been described and utilized in various aspects of foot and ankle surgery over the past several decades. In regards to ankle surgery, flexible fixation devices have been used for stabilization of the ankle syndesmosis as well as augmentation of lateral collateral ankle ligament repair. In the foot, flexible fixation devices have been incorporated into hallux valgus or varus correction, Lisfranc injury repair, and more recently spring ligament repair augmentation. This article reviews the various applications for flexible fixation in foot and ankle surgery, as well as evidence-based literature on surgical applications and clinical outcomes.

FLEXIBLE FIXATION APPLICATIONS AND ANKLE SURGERY

Flexible fixation, for purposes of this article, will refer to implant devices that are flexible (ie, suture-button or suture-tape) rather than rigid (ie, metal screws).

Disclosures: K.M. Raspovic is a consultant for Orthofix. The rest of the authors have nothing to disclose.
Department of Orthopaedic Surgery, UT Southwestern Medical Center, 1801 Inwood Road, Dallas, Texas 75390, USA
* Corresponding author.
E-mail address: Katherine.Raspovic@utsouthwestern.edu

FLEXIBLE FIXATION OF THE ANKLE SYNDESMOSIS

Perhaps the most common use of flexible fixation in foot and ankle surgery is the utilization of suture-button implant devices for injuries of the ankle syndesmosis (**Figs. 1 and 2**). The distal tibiofibular syndesmosis consists of the anterior inferior tibiofibular, posterior interior tibiofibular, transverse tibiofibular, and interosseous ligaments.[1] This ligamentous complex stabilizes the distal fibula against the fibular incisura of the distal tibia.[1] Disruption of the syndesmosis occurs in roughly 13% of ankle fracture injuries.[2–4] Injury of the syndesmosis is also associated with high ankle sprains and the Maisonneuve fracture (fibular neck). The goal of syndesmotic repair is to restore the anatomic alignment of the distal fibula and the fibular incisura of the tibia. Misdiagnosis or inadequate reduction may result in persistent pain and acceleration of the development of osteoarthritis of the tibiotalar joint. Surgical repair of the syndesmosis may consist of either rigid screw fixation or fixation with a flexible suture-button device. Screw fixation has been the traditional treatment for surgical repair of syndesmotic injuries; however, the use of suture-button devices has increased in popularity over the past decade. One of the earliest studies on suture-button fixation of the syndesmosis was published by Thornes and colleagues[5] in 2003. This cadaveric study compared fixation of a syndesmotic injury with a suture-button device versus fixation with a single tetracortical 4.5 mm screw. In this biomechanical study, the suture-button was found to perform equally to standard screw fixation.[5] In 2005, Thornes and colleagues[6] introduced suture-button fixation for ankle fractures with concomitant syndesmotic injury in a prospective study comparing suture-button fixation with screw fixation.[6] In this first clinical study, patients who underwent suture-button fixation had significantly better American Orthopaedic Food & Ankle Society (AOFAS) scores at 3 and 12 months postoperatively, faster return to work, and no need for implant removal when compared with the patients who underwent screw fixation.[6] The suture-button construct in the 2005 Thornes and colleagues[6] study consisted of a #5 braided polyester suture. This braided suture was looped twice through the center holes of 2 endobuttons; pulling the suture ends allows for tightening of the buttons together, reducing the syndesmosis.[6] Since that time, flexible syndesmotic fixation has evolved, with multiple devices commercially available for use (GRAVITY SYNCHFIX Syndesmotic Fixation Device, 2018 Wright Medical Group; Syndesmosis TightRope, Arthrex, Inc., Naples, FL; Invisiknot, Smith and Nephew, Inc.; ZipTight, Zimmer Biomet).

Complications of screw fixation of the syndesmosis include screw failure, need for screw removal necessitating a return to the operating room, and potentially loss of syndesmotic reduction after screw removal.[7] Use of suture-button fixation for repair of a syndesmotic injury may allow for a reduced rate of implant removal and potentially less likely recurrence of syndesmotic instability.[8] Another benefit of suture-button fixation is that it allows for physiologic motion of the distal fibula in relation to the tibia, whereas a screw construct is rigid.[9] Additional clinical studies have compared the use of screw versus suture-button devices. Recently, a prospective, randomized, multicenter study compared the clinical outcomes of patients treated with either a suture-button implant or screw fixation of an acute syndesmotic disruption.[10] Patients who underwent repair of an acute rupture of the ankle syndesmosis were randomized into either the dynamic fixation (flexible/suture-button) group or the static fixation (rigid/screw) group. Seventy patients were initially enrolled. Five patients were lost to follow up. Ultimately, 65 patients were available for follow-up including 33 patients in the dynamic group and 32 patients in the static fixation group. Static (rigid/screw) fixation consisted of one 3.5 mm cortical screw spanning 4 cortices. The dynamic (flexible) group underwent suture-button fixation (TightRope, Arthrex Inc., Naples, FL).

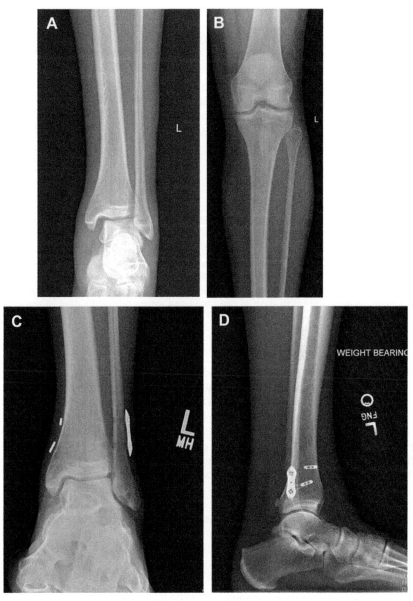

Fig. 1. 48-year-old active male with left fibular neck fracture/syndesmotic disruption after a fall. (*A*) AP radiograph of the left ankle demonstrating medial clear space widening. (*B*) Radiograph of the left knee/proximal tibia and fibula showing a fibular neck fracture. (*C*) AP postoperative weightbearing ankle radiograph demonstrating reduction and fixation of the syndesmotic injury with 2 suture-button devices. (*D*) Lateral post-operative radiograph demonstrating fixation of syndesmosis with 2 suture-button devices and a lateral plate.

Postoperative treatment protocol for all patients in both groups consisted of non-weightbearing for 6 weeks followed by physical therapy. A higher implant failure rate in the static fixation (rigid/screw) group was found compared with the dynamic (flexible/suture-button) group (36.1% vs 0%, $P<.05$). Loss of reduction occurred in 4 cases,

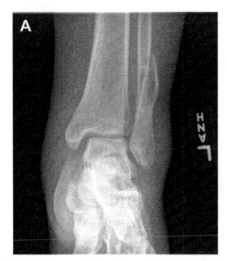 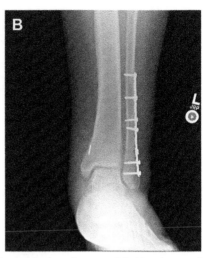

Fig. 2. 16-year-old healthy male with bimalleolar equivalent fracture. (A) AP preoperative radiograph demonstrating a distal fibular fracture, widening of the medial clear space, and decreased overlap of the distal tibia and fibula. (B) Postoperative radiograph after open reduction and internal fixation of the fibula and suture-button fixation of the syndesmotic injury.

all of which were in the static fixation (rigid/screw) group (11.1% vs 0%, P=.06).[10] A recent systematic review identified 10 studies with a total of 390 patients who sustained distal tibiofibular syndesmosis injury.[7] This review compared patients who underwent surgical treatment with traditional screw fixation to patients who underwent suture-button fixation. Overall, the suture-button patients had similar postoperative outcomes as measured by AOFAS scores, and similar postoperative complication rates when compared with patients undergoing screw fixation. Patients who underwent suture-button fixation had better objective tibiotalar joint range of motion, earlier return to work, lower rate of implant removal, and lower rate of implant failure. The studies in this review that reported the rate of malreduction had a lower rate of malreduction using the suture-button (1%) compared with traditional screw fixation (12.6%).[7] Although both methods of fixation are widely used, suture-button fixation may have several benefits as discussed previously, compared with screw fixation of the distal tibiofibular syndesmosis.

FLEXIBLE FIXATION AND LATERAL ANKLE STABILIZATION

The use of flexible fixation for augmentation of lateral collateral ankle ligament repair has increased in popularity over the past several years. Suture-tape augmentation has been used to help improve stability when performing a Bröstrom procedure of the anterior talofibular ligament (ATFL). Bröstrom originally described an anatomic suture repair of the ATFL in the 1960s.[11] Since then there have been multiple variations of this direct suture repair to include the use of bone anchors and suture-tape to augment the repair and increase overall stability. The InternalBrace (Arthrex Inc., Naples, FL) is an example of a system designed to augment the lateral ankle ligament repair and consists of osseous anchors and suture-tape (BioComposite SwiveLock suture anchors, FiberTape, Arthrex Inc., Naples, FL). Watson and Lamour[12] described the original technique using InternalBrace in 2015. They described their technique as a "knotless, suture anchor-based system that can increase the ligament repair construct strength to 250 N, which is 1.6-times greater than the native ATFL and 3.7 times greater than the traditional Bröstrom repair." The benefits of this construct are earlier return to activity and decreased rate of recurrent instability.[12]

Viens and colleagues[13] performed the first biomechanical cadaveric study comparing 3 groups: intact ATFL, suture-tape augmentation alone, and Bröstrom repair plus suture-tape augmentation.[13] They found that augmentation with suture-tape alone had a 50% higher load to failure and stiffness compared with an intact ATFL. They also showed that suture-tape augmentation alone or Bröstrom repair plus suture-tape augmentation resulted in a stronger construct compared with a standard Bröstrom repair.[13] Another cadaveric study compared 3 groups undergoing different ATFL reconstruction techniques: the traditional Bröstrom technique, repair with suture anchors, and suture anchor combined with suture-tape augmentation.[14] The suture anchor combined with suture-tape augmentation technique had a statistically higher angle at failure and higher maximum torque at failure compared with the other 2 techniques.[14] Although these were cadaveric studies, augmentation of the Bröstrom with suture-tape demonstrated improved stability from a biomechanical standpoint.[13,14] A retrospective case series of 81 patients undergoing a Bröstrom repair augmented with suture-tape showed satisfactory outcomes at a mean follow-up of 11.5 months.[15] Sixty-seven percent of patients were brace-free and returned to sport activity.[15] Another retrospective study of patients undergoing a modified Bröstrom repair augmented with suture-tape for ankle instability caused by generalized laxity found significant clinical improvement at a mean follow-up of 2 years.[16] A 2016 study demonstrated a faster return to sports and activity in patients undergoing modified Bröstrom repair with suture-tape augmentation compared with patients undergoing modified Bröstrom only without the augmentation.[17] Suture-tape augmentation has also been studied in revision procedures. A recent review of patients undergoing a revision modified Bröstrom procedure augmented with suture-tape revealed significant clinical improvement at a mean follow-up of 38.5 months.[18] Although more long-term studies are needed, augmentation of the Bröstrom repair with suture-tape has demonstrated improved strength of repair and good clinical outcomes.

FLEXIBLE FIXATION APPLICATIONS IN THE FOREFOOT, MIDFOOT, AND HINDFOOT
Lisfranc Suture-Button Applications

Anatomic reduction is the key to successful outcomes when surgically treating Lisfranc injuries (**Fig. 3**).[19] Disruption of the Lisfranc ligament and resulting diastasis has traditionally been treated with screw fixation and/or plate fixation. Potential disadvantages of screw fixation include hardware failure, need for removal, and articular damage when performing open reduction and internal fixation (ORIF) of this injury if transosseous screws are used. Lisfranc injuries include a broad spectrum; they range from sprain, to subluxation, to fracture and fracture/dislocation.[20,21] Arthrodesis versus ORIF of the Lisfranc complex is an area of debate beyond the scope of this article. Stabilization of the Lisfranc ligament disruption and resulting diastasis with a suture-button device was introduced by Cottom and colleagues[22] in 2008, reporting on 3 cases. The authors selected this method of fixation for several reasons. First, the implant is less likely to break compared to a screw; additionally, it may be left intact, which helps to avoid a return to the operating room, and it allows for micromotion as would a normal Lisfranc ligament. All patients had satisfactory outcomes in the short term.[22]

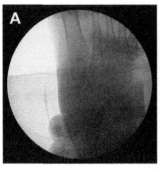
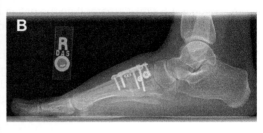
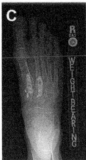

Fig. 3. 24-year-old healthy woman with right foot Lisfranc fracture dislocation involving the first and second tarsometatarsal joints. (*A*) Intraoperative stress view of the right foot showing diastasis caused by disruption of the Lisfranc ligament. (*B*) Lateral and (*C*) AP weightbearing postoperative radiographs showing successful open reduction and internal fixation of the first and second tarsometatarsal joints with bridge plating and suture-button fixation of the Lisfranc ligamentous disruption.

The strength of a suture-button construct for Lisfranc ligament repair has been evaluated in several studies. A biomechanical study in 2009 compared the stability of a cannulated screw with a suture-button construct for stabilization of Lisfranc ligamentous injury and diastasis.[23] The Lisfranc ligament was transected in 14 cadavers. Fixation was then performed with either a cannulated screw or a suture-button construct. Stability was found to be similar between the 2 different methods of fixation.[23] A second cadaveric study performed in 2010 also compared traditional screw fixation with suture-button fixation and found that screw fixation had less displacement under an axial load compared with suture-button fixation.[24]

Surgical outcomes in athletes have been evaluated in several studies using suture-button repair of Lisfranc injuries. A recent retrospective review evaluated the outcome of surgical treatment of chronic Lisfranc injury in professional dancers and high-level athletes.[25] This was a small series of 7 patients who had failed conservative treatment after late presentation. All patients returned to their full activity level by 6 months after surgery, and average AOFAS scores improved from 65 preoperatively to 97 postoperatively at a mean follow-up of 15 months.[25] In another small series, 5 professional soccer and rugby players underwent open reduction and suture-button fixation of a Lisfranc injury.[26] The average time to return to full competition was 20.4 weeks, and all patients in the study returned to elite sporting activity.[26] Although larger surgical series with long-term outcomes are still needed, suture-button fixation in the properly selected, active patient appears to have good clinical outcomes. Potential advantages compared with screw fixation may include the avoidance of an additional surgical procedure for removal and less chance of construct failure. Earlier return to sport activity and preservation of micromotion are additional potential benefits of this construct.

Hallux Valgus Suture-Button Applications

Although it is not a common treatment for surgical correction of hallux abducto valgus, suture-button fixation has been described for correction in several small series. The authors of this current review prefer correction of hallux abducto valgus deformity with osteotomies or a Lapidus procedure; however, it is worthwhile to note that one may utilize a suture-button device to aid in the reduction of the first and second intermetatarsal angle (IMA). A small series (5 patients) showed a statistically significant reduction in IMA at intermediate and long-term follow up using a suture-button device (Arthrex Mini TightRope); however, 60% of patients required surgical revision.[27] A retrospective review of 14 cases showed postoperative improvement of IMA and hallux valgus angle; however, the mean follow-up was only 6 months.[28] Another retrospective case series of 25 patients (mean follow-up of 22.5 months) demonstrated significant improvement in the IMA and hallux valgus angles ($P<.05$); however, 8 patients (32%) developed a second metatarsal stress fracture.[29] Fracture of the second metatarsal has also been reported by others when using this technique.[30,31] Although using a suture-button may help avoid osteotomy and therefore decrease postoperative recovery time, studies supporting the use of this in hallux abducto valgus surgical correction are limited.

Hallux Varus Suture-Button Applications

The use of suture-button fixation may have a role in the treatment of flexible hallux varus, although there are only a few reports. Gerbert and colleagues[32] presented a case report using a suture-button construct for correction of an acquired hallux varus. Interestingly, the patient had previously undergone a McBride bunionectomy with a closing wedge osteotomy of the first metatarsal base 15 years prior, and had only noticed symptoms and varus alignment 2 years prior to presentation. Prior to the corrective hallux varus surgery, the patient had full and pain-free range of motion of the first metatarsophalangeal joint and an abnormally low IM angle. She underwent correction of the hallux varus with suture-button fixation and returned to full activity at 10 months after surgery.[32] Barp and colleagues[33] reported on a single case of hallux varus after adductor hallucis tendon rupture, treated with suture-button fixation. At 3-year follow-up, the patient had maintained surgical correction and was pain free.[33] Further studies are needed on the use of suture-button fixation for hallux varus repair; however, it may be a useful tool to aid in correction of a flexible hallux varus deformity.

Spring Ligament Applications

Disruption or insufficiency of the calcaneonavicular (spring) ligament has been shown to result in peritalar subluxation of the talonavicular joint.[34] A unique technique for augmentation of the spring ligament was introduced by Acevedo and Vora in 2013.[35] They described a primary repair of the ligament with augmentation using suture-tape and bone anchors (FiberTape and Swivel Lock anchors, Arthrex Inc., Naples, FL) in conjunction with other flexible flatfoot/stage 2 posterior tibial tendon dysfunction (PTTD) reconstruction procedures.[35] The suture-tape replicates the superomedial and inferomedial bands of the spring ligament.[35] Their reconstruction included removal of the nonviable posterior tibial tendon, harvest of the flexor digitorum longus (FDL) tendon, completion of necessary osseous extra-articular procedures, repair of the spring ligament, suture-tape augmentation of the spring ligament, and then transfer of the FDL tendon. The proximal limb of the suture-tape augmentation is secured into the sustentaculum tali with an anchor. The proximal limb then divides into 2 separate limbs to recreate the superomedial and inferomedial bands. The superomedial band is replicated by advancing the first limb of the suture-tape from dorsal to plantar through a bone tunnel in the medial aspect of the navicular. The inferomedial band is made by advancing the second limb of the suture-tape through the bone tunnel from plantar to dorsal navicular with the FDL tendon. A biotenodesis screw is then inserted into the navicular while the suture-tape limbs and FDL tendon are placed under tension.[35]

A recent biomechanical study by Aynardi and colleagues[36] compared the strength of spring ligament suture repair (control group) to spring ligament repair augmented with suture-tape (FiberTape/InternalBrace, Arthrex, Inc., Naples, FL) in a cadaver model. All specimens underwent flatfoot creation and reconstruction. After cyclic loading, all specimens in the control group (spring ligament suture repair) failed (8/8) compared with 1 of 8 that failed in the study group (repair with suture-tape augmentation).[36] Although more studies are necessary to show the long-term benefits and outcomes, suture-tape augmentation of a spring ligament repair, in conjunction with the other procedures required of a stage 2 PTTD flatfoot correction, may provide increased stability and help prevent recurrence of peritalar subluxation.

SUMMARY

Flexible fixation continues to evolve and increase in popularity in foot and ankle surgery. Flexible fixation devices are often used for stabilization of the ankle syndesmosis and for augmentation of lateral collateral ankle ligament injury repairs. Flexible fixation has been used in hallux valgus or varus correction, as well as Lisfranc injury repair, although clinical studies for use in these scenarios are limited. More recently, spring ligament repair augmentation has been described in flexible flatfoot reconstructive procedures. Possible benefits of flexible fixation may include less need for removal, allowance of physiologic micromotion, and improved strength when used for augmentation of ligamentous repairs. Although further clinical studies are needed to assess the long-term outcomes, the utilization of these devices will likely continue to increase in foot and ankle surgery as surgeons continue to develop methods to improve patient satisfaction and overall outcomes.

REFERENCES

1. Liu GT, Ryan E, Gustafson E, et al. Three-dimensional computed tomographic characterization of normal anatomic morphology and variations of the distal tibiofibular syndesmosis. J Foot Ankle Surg 2018;57(6):1130–6.
2. Dattani R, Patnaik S, Kantak A, et al. Injuries to the tibiofibular syndesmosis. J Bone Joint Surg Br 2008;90(4):405–10.
3. Lindsjo U. Operative treatment of ankle fractures. Acta Orthop Scand Suppl 1981;189:1–131.
4. Vosseller JT, Karl JW, Greisberg JK. Incidence of syndesmotic injury. Orthopedics 2014;37(3):e226–9.
5. Thornes B, Walsh A, Hislop M, et al. Suture-endobutton fixation of ankle tibiofibular diastasis: a cadaver study. Foot Ankle Int 2003;24(2):142–6.
6. Thornes B, Shannon F, Guiney AM, et al. Suture-button syndesmosis fixation: accelerated rehabilitation and improved outcomes. Clin Orthop Relat Res 2005;(431):207–12.

7. Zhang P, Liang Y, He J, et al. A systematic review of suture-button versus syndesmotic screw in the treatment of distal tibiofibular syndesmosis injury. BMC Musculoskelet Disord 2017;18(1):286.

8. Naqvi GA, Cunningham P, Lynch B, et al. Fixation of ankle syndesmotic injuries: comparison of tightrope fixation and syndesmotic screw fixation for accuracy of syndesmotic reduction. Am J Sports Med 2012;40(12):2828–35.

9. Scranton PE Jr, McMaster JG, Kelly E. Dynamic fibular function: a new concept. Clin Orthop Relat Res 1976;(118):76–81.

10. Laflamme M, Belzile EL, Bédard L, et al. A prospective randomized multicenter trial comparing clinical outcomes of patients treated surgically with a static or dynamic implant for acute ankle syndesmosis rupture. J Orthop Trauma 2015;29(5): 216–23.

11. Brostrom L. Sprained ankles. VI. Surgical treatment of "chronic" ligament ruptures. Acta Chir Scand 1966;132(5):551–65.

12. Waston TSAL, Richard J. Open modified Broström ankle reconstruction with internal brace augmentation: a novel approach. Orthopedics Today 2015.

13. Viens NA, Wijdicks CA, Campbell KJ, et al. Anterior talofibular ligament ruptures, part 1: biomechanical comparison of augmented Brostrom repair techniques with the intact anterior talofibular ligament. Am J Sports Med 2014;42(2):405–11.

14. Schuh R, Benca E, Willegger M, et al. Comparison of Brostrom technique, suture anchor repair, and tape augmentation for reconstruction of the anterior talofibular ligament. Knee Surg Sports Traumatol Arthrosc 2016;24(4):1101–7.

15. Coetzee JC, Ellington JK, Ronan JA, et al. Functional results of open Brostrom ankle ligament repair augmented with a suture tape. Foot Ankle Int 2018;39(3): 304–10.

16. Cho BK, Park KJ, Park JK, et al. Outcomes of the modified Brostrom procedure augmented with suture-tape for ankle instability in patients with generalized ligamentous laxity. Foot Ankle Int 2017;38(4):405–11.

17. Yoo JS, Yang EA. Clinical results of an arthroscopic modified Brostrom operation with and without an internal brace. J Orthop Traumatol 2016;17(4):353–60.

18. Cho BK, Kim YM, Choi SM, et al. Revision anatomical reconstruction of the lateral ligaments of the ankle augmented with suture tape for patients with a failed Brostrom procedure. Bone Joint J 2017;99-B(9):1183–9.

19. Kuo RS, Tejwani NC, Digiovanni CW, et al. Outcome after open reduction and internal fixation of Lisfranc joint injuries. J Bone Joint Surg Am 2000;82-A(11): 1609–18.

20. Welck MJ, Zinchenko R, Rudge B. Lisfranc injuries. Injury 2015;46(4):536–41.

21. Mulcahy H. Lisfranc injury: current concepts. Radiol Clin North Am 2018;56(6): 859–76.

22. Cottom JM, Hyer CF, Berlet GC. Treatment of Lisfranc fracture dislocations with an interosseous suture button technique: a review of 3 cases. J Foot Ankle Surg 2008;47(3):250–8.

23. Panchbhavi VK, Vallurupalli S, Yang J, et al. Screw fixation compared with suture-button fixation of isolated Lisfranc ligament injuries. J Bone Joint Surg Am 2009; 91(5):1143–8.

24. Ahmed S, Bolt B, McBryde A. Comparison of standard screw fixation versus suture button fixation in Lisfranc ligament injuries. Foot Ankle Int 2010;31(10):892–6.

25. Charlton T, Boe C, Thordarson DB. Suture button fixation treatment of chronic Lisfranc injury in professional dancers and high-level athletes. J Dance Med Sci 2015;19(4):135–9.

26. Jain K, Drampalos E, Clough TM. Results of suture button fixation with targeting device aid for displaced ligamentous Lisfranc injuries in the elite athlete. Foot (Edinb) 2017;30:43–6.
27. Ponnapula P, Wittock R. Application of an interosseous suture and button device for hallux valgus correction: a review of outcomes in a small series. J Foot Ankle Surg 2010;49(2):159.e21-6.
28. Holmes GB Jr, Hsu AR. Correction of intermetatarsal angle in hallux valgus using small suture button device. Foot Ankle Int 2013;34(4):543–9.
29. Weatherall JM, Chapman CB, Shapiro SL. Postoperative second metatarsal fractures associated with suture-button implant in hallux valgus surgery. Foot Ankle Int 2013;34(1):104–10.
30. Mader DW, Han NM. Bilateral second metatarsal stress fractures after hallux valgus correction with the use of a tension wire and button fixation system. J Foot Ankle Surg 2010;49(5):488.e15-9.
31. Kemp TJ, Hirose CB, Coughlin MJ. Fracture of the second metatarsal following suture button fixation device in the correction of hallux valgus. Foot Ankle Int 2010;31(8):712–6.
32. Gerbert J, Traynor C, Blue K, et al. Use of the Mini TightRope(R) for correction of hallux varus deformity. J Foot Ankle Surg 2011;50(2):245–51.
33. Barp EA, Temple EW, Hall JL, et al. Treatment of hallux varus after traumatic adductor hallucis tendon rupture. J Foot Ankle Surg 2018;57(2):418–20.
34. Jennings MM, Christensen JC. The effects of sectioning the spring ligament on rearfoot stability and posterior tibial tendon efficiency. J Foot Ankle Surg 2008; 47(3):219–24.
35. Acevedo J, Vora A. Anatomical reconstruction of the spring ligament complex: "internal brace" augmentation. Foot Ankle Spec 2013;6(6):441–5.
36. Aynardi MC, Saloky K, Roush EP, et al. Biomechanical evaluation of spring ligament augmentation with the FiberTape device in a cadaveric flatfoot model. Foot Ankle Int 2019;40(5):596–602.

Amnion Applications in the Foot and Ankle

Thanh Dinh, DPM*, Casey Lewis, DPM

KEYWORDS

• Amnion • Chorion • Foot and ankle • Wound healing • Surgical applications

KEY POINTS

- Amnion and chorion products show great promise and have real potential to be mainstays of treatment for chronic, nonhealing wounds.
- Although amniotic products do carry a cost, the decrease in time to healing, with the assumed subsequent decrease in complication and infection rates, should also be taken into consideration.
- These products, with their unique biologic potential and availability in the clinical setting, may prove to be beneficial in a vast array of podiatric surgical applications.

INTRODUCTION

Over the last decade, the therapeutic benefits of amniotic tissue have been intensely studied because of the promise of tissue regeneration secondary to the abundance of growth factors, cytokines, and matrix components inherent in its tissue origin. In addition to the vast regenerative profile, downregulation of inflammatory factors and lack of an immunogenic response results confer several advantages in many clinical settings. Furthermore, the decreased inflammation has been observed to result in minimal to no scarring and graft rejection.

With improvements in methods of sterilization, processing, and storage capabilities, these tissues are becoming increasingly available in the clinical domain and more commonplace in wound healing and tissue regeneration applications.[1] Compared with other biologic tissue grafts, the expanded shelf life has allowed for growth in use in many medical specialties, including ophthalmology, general surgery, plastic surgery, and orthopedic surgery.[2]

Amniotic tissue consists of 2 distinct components: the inner amniotic membrane and the outer chorionic membrane that is in contact with the maternal tissue in utero. The amniotic membrane supports the development of the fetus during pregnancy and

Disclosure Statement: The authors have nothing to disclose.
Department of Surgery, Division of Podiatry, Beth Israel Deaconess Medical Center, Harvard Medical School, 1 Deaconess Road, Boston, MA 02215, USA
* Corresponding author.
E-mail address: tdinh@bidmc.harvard.edu

has received significant research attention because of its ability to repair tissue directly through the efforts of the extracellular matrix, composed of collagen, fibronectin, laminin and abundance of growth factors and cytokines. The amniotic membrane is a tissue of particular interest as a source of readily available multipotent stem cells and factors that promote tissue renewal[3] (**Fig. 1**).

Composed of a thin epithelial layer, a thick basement membrane, and an avascular stroma, the amniotic membrane contains collagen types III, IV, V, and VII, as well as fibronectin and laminin. The presence of fibroblasts and growth factors yields the unique properties such as the ability to suppress fibrosis, prevent bacteria proliferation, and promote wound healing.[4] The amniotic membrane contains 2 cell types of different embryologic origin, specifically amnion epithelial cells, derived from the embryonic ectoderm, and amnion mesenchymal cells, derived from embryonic mesoderm.[5] Owing to its embryologic origin, amniotic membrane acts as a nonimmunogenic agent allowing for transplantation without risk of rejection in clinical applications.[6,7] This lack of immunogenic response and rejection following human amniotic tissue transplantation into human volunteers has been demonstrated.[8]

ANTI-INFLAMMATORY PROPERTIES

Inflammation is the initial and critical stage of the wound healing process. However, prolonged inflammation has been attributed as the root cause of chronic, nonhealing wounds in addition to promoting scar formation. Interestingly, observation of fetal wound healing has exhibited minimal inflammation because of an increased persistence on the regenerative stage of the wound healing cascade.[9] The endurance of the regenerative stage in fetal wound healing is in stark contrast to the prolonged inflammation observed in adult wound healing leading to scarring.[10] Although the exact pathways remain unknown, research has shed light on several factors responsible for the anti-inflammatory properties inherent in amniotic tissue, namely the presence of various growth factors and cytokines.

At the molecular level, amniotic tissue has been identified as possessing an abundance of interleukin-10 (IL-10), which has been shown to reduce scarring through its inhibition of IL-6. IL-6 is known to stimulate keratinocyte migration and proliferation, along with the stimulation of fibroblast proliferation and angiogenesis, processes that contribute to scarring.[11] Evidence of the role of IL-6 in diminished scar formation was provided by Liechty and colleagues,[12] who demonstrated decreased levels of IL-

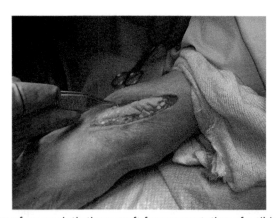

Fig. 1. Application of an amniotic tissue graft for augmentation of a tibialis tendon repair.

6 in fetal wounds compared with adult wounds and that supplementation with IL-6 resulted in increased scar formation.

Decreased inflammation observed in amniotic tissue has also been speculated to be the result of innate suppression of the transforming growth factor-β (TGF-β) signaling system.[13] The TGF-β system is a critical part of inflammation, fibroblast proliferation, angiogenesis, collagen synthesis and deposition, and extracellular matrix remodeling.[14] When amniotic membrane was used on human corneal cells, decreased TGF-β signaling, DNA synthesis, and myofibroblast differentiation was observed.[15] The role of TGF-β signaling in the role of inflammation and scar formation is further supported by a study indicating a deficiency of TGF-β1 in fetal skin compared with adult skin, as well as the observation that supplementation with exogenous TGF-β1 resulted in increased inflammation and scar formation.[16]

In addition to increased expression of IL-10 and suppression of TGF-β signaling, amniotic tissue possesses a profusion of high-molecular-weight hyaluronic acid (HA), thought to inhibit collagen deposition to prevent fibrotic tissue formation.[11,17] In contrast, adult tissues are composed of greater quantities of low-molecular-weight HA, which promotes inflammation and has a deleterious effect on wound healing.[18] HA helps limit inflammation through the suppression of certain matrix metalloproteinases, and it also suppresses the fibrinolytic activity mediated by the urokinase-type plasminogen activator and urokinase-type receptor systems, resulting in decreased inflammation.[19]

PROCESSING AND STORAGE

Fresh amniotic membrane tissue is typically harvested during scheduled Cesarean sections from donors who have undergone rigorous screening for infectious diseases. Fresh grafts require immediate transplantation, and thus preservation techniques such as cryopreservation or dehydration have been utilized to increase storage time to allow for delayed clinical applications of the tissue.[20] Although both cryopreservation and dehydration techniques have exhibited diminished maximum loads to failure compared with fresh tissue, both retained their tensile strength and also their ability to promote the proliferation of dermal fibroblasts for wound healing.[21]

CLINICAL APPLICATIONS IN FOOT AND ANKLE SURGERY

Amniotic membrane tissue has been increasingly studied for its tissue regeneration properties in foot and ankle surgery. Current areas of investigation include plantar fasciitis, ligament and tendon healing, cartilage restoration, and wound healing. In vivo studies have found that amniotic membrane may increase collagen production, facilitating the repair of tendons and other soft tissue structures.[22] Additionally, the use of amniotic membrane may reduce the fibrosis and adhesion formation commonly complicating tendon surgery.[23]

As a result of the promising early results with amniotic tissue augmentation, researchers have taken the opportunity to pursue the use of this regenerative treatment in other clinical scenarios. In 1 novel study, Anderson and Swayzee[24] published a series of 101 patients who underwent ankle arthroscopy with microfracture for treatment of osteochondral lesions of the talus. Among those 101 patients, 54 had augmentation with AM suspension allograft. When compared with those patients who did not have augmentation, patients whose surgeries were augmented with AM had improved pain and functional outcome scores at early and 24-month follow-ups.

PLANTAR FASCIITIS

Plantar fasciitis is a common condition, with an estimated 1 million outpatient visits annually.[25] Plantar fasciitis is frequently described as a chronic inflammatory condition; however, histopathologic studies evaluating the plantar fascia ligament in patients with plantar fasciitis demonstrate collagen degeneration and disorientation. Additionally, there is an absence of inflammatory cells, suggesting a more degenerative process similar to tendinopathy.[26] As a result, researchers have hypothesized that growth amniotic tissue providing growth factors may provide benefit as a treatment for tendinopathies with the potential to reverse the degenerative process and encourage the regeneration of healthy tendon.[27]

In a pilot study, the efficacy of cryopreserved human amniotic membrane (c-hAM) injection compared with corticosteroid injection was evaluated for the treatment of plantar fasciitis.[28] Patients were randomized into one of 2 treatment groups: c-hAM or corticosteroid. Patients received an injection at their initial baseline visit with an option for a second injection at their first 6-week follow-up. Total follow-up was obtained for 12 weeks after the most recent injection. The primary outcome measurement was the Foot Health Status Questionnaire (FHSQ). The secondary outcome measurements were the Visual Analog Scale (VAS) and verbally reported percentage improvement. Data were analyzed between groups for the 2 different cohorts (1 injection vs 2 injections). Twenty-three patients had complete follow-up. Fourteen patients were randomized to receive corticosteroid, and 9 patients were randomized to receive c-hAM. The authors concluded that cryopreserved c-hAM injection may be safe and comparable to corticosteroid injection for treatment of plantar fasciitis but required further investigation.

To further investigate the benefits of amniotic tissue in plantar fasciitis, in a prospective, single-blinded, randomized controlled multicenter trial, patients diagnosed with plantar fasciitis were randomized to receive a micronized dehydrated amniotic membrane injection (treatment group) or a 0.9% sodium chloride placebo injection (placebo group).[29] The primary efficacy endpoint was change in visual analog scale (VAS) score for pain between baseline and the 3-month follow-up visit. At baseline, VAS scores were similar for treatment and control subjects ($P = .8347$). At the 3-month follow-up visit, the mean VAS scores in the treatment group were 76% lower compared with a 45% reduction in mean VAS scores for controls, which equated to a 54-point drop in the treatment group compared with a 32-point drop in the control group ($P<.0001$). Overall, at the 3-month study visit, 60 (82.2%) of subjects in the treatment group, and 34 (47.2%) of subjects in the control group reported at least a 50% reduction in VAS score from baseline ($P<.0001$).

TENDON REPAIR AUGMENTATION

As a result of its ability to repair and regenerate tissue, amniotic applications in tendon regeneration have been investigated, but mostly in the animal studies. In a sheep Achilles tendon model, amniotic epithelial cells (AECs) were transplanted into experimentally induced Achilles tendon defects to evaluate tendon regeneration potential and the underlying mechanisms involved.[30] Evaluation of the in situ tissue repair revealed that the AEC-treated tendons had improved structural and mechanical properties compared with the non AEC-treated tendons during the early phase of healing.

Furthermore, immunohistochemical and biochemical analyses indicated that the extracellular matrix remodeling in the AEC-treated tendons was more rapid with the immature collagen fibers replaced by mature fibers in 28 days. Through spatial–temporal analysis of cellularity, proliferation index, vascular area, and leukocyte infiltration, it was observed that the injected AECs rapidly migrated initially to healthy tissue. This then progressed to a centripetal healing process, with gradual advancement to the core of the lesion.

It was postulated that this peculiar healing pattern was induced by the growth factor stimulatory influence of TGF-β1 and VEGF in addition to host progenitor cell recruitment. Additionally, the direct tenogenic AEC differentiation resulted in the regeneration of a new tendon matrix. These findings demonstrated the premise that AECs can support tendon regeneration, and their regenerative effects on growth factor expression may be used to develop future strategies to treat tendon disease.

Similarly, Ozgenel and colleagues[31] found favorable results in flexor tendon repair treated with human amniotic fluid (HAF) in a rabbit model. The HAF-injected tendon injuries showed improved mechanical strength and elasticity when compared with the placebo group injected with saline. In addition to improved healing, the investigators also noted that at 12 weeks, the tendons treated with HAF showed decreased adhesions compared with repairs in the placebo group. By 20 weeks, HAF-treated tendons had higher tensile load values compared with the control group.

Although some animal investigations have demonstrated improved healing and decreased adhesions with amniotic tissue supplementation, other studies have found minimal benefits to their use. In fact, the use of amniotic tissue may not be the only tissue capable of promoting collagen regeneration and inhibition of inflammatory cytokines. In 1 study, the effect of tissue augmentation on Achilles tendon healing with small intestinal submucosa (SIS) compared with human amniotic membrane (HAM) was investigated in a rabbit model.[32] A total of 48 New Zealand white rabbits had full-thickness transverse tenotomies made on the right leg, and the laceration site was subsequently wrapped with HAM or SIS. Histologic evaluation was performed to identify expression of collagen I and levels of inflammatory cytokines IL-1β, IL-6, and TNF-α. Additionally, adhesion formation was evaluated.

The investigators found that were no significant differences in filamentous adhesion, cross-sectional areas of the laceration sites, levels of inflammatory response, and collagen type I expression between the HAM- and SIS-treated groups. However, they found that the SIS-treated group showed superior biomechanical properties and neovascularization compared with the HAM-treated group in the early stage of healing at day 7 and day 14 of healing. The authors concluded that SIS augmentation in the treatment of Achilles tendon injury in a rabbit model showed superior biomechanical properties and neovascularization over HAM-treated tendons.

Although some animal investigations demonstrated improved healing with amniotic tissue supplementation, others have demonstrated no benefits. Coban and colleagues[33] evaluated 72 Achilles tendon repairs, with 24 receiving amniotic fluid injection, 24 receiving a membrane wrap, and 24 receiving no added treatment following suture repair of the tendon. The tendons were evaluated histopathologically at weeks 1 and 2 and biomechanically at week 3 with no difference in healing time or strength or repair. The only statistical differences were minor histopathological changes that did not confer any mechanical advantages.

WOUND HEALING

By far the most well-known indication for amniotic tissue products is focused on wound-healing applications. Delayed wound healing presents a significant personal burden to patients and a challenge for providers, with a significant cost to the health care system. The treatment of chronic wounds including diabetic foot ulcers alone has been estimated between $6.2 and 18.7 billion annually, with the vast majority of these costs occurring in the outpatient setting.[34] Patients with chronic wounds are often monitored closely to mitigate the risk of complications such as infection leading to the more devastating complications of osteomyelitis and subsequent amputations. The widespread impact of chronic wounds has providers seeking alternative, adjunctive treatments in order to improve care for their patients, and ultimately achieve complete and continued wound closure.

Comorbidities such as diabetes mellitus, peripheral arterial disease, and a diminished immune response can complicate the wound healing process, resulting in the search for novel treatments to address these hurdles. Because of the observation that chronic wounds have stalled in the wound healing process, current guidelines for the treatment of diabetic ulcers advocate that wounds that fail to achieve a 40% reduction in ulcer size after 4 weeks of treatment should be considered for more advanced treatment modalities.[35] Although advanced wound care products do carry an increased cost in the short term, they can play a critical role in stimulating the healing process and reducing longer-term costs and complications.[36] Amniotic tissue in particular has been proposed as an ideal therapy given the regenerative benefits, and the efficacy of these therapies has been investigated in several clinical studies, with promising results demonstrated.

MECHANISMS OF ACTION

Preliminary studies have suggested that amniotic tissue aids wound healing through a variety of methods, including antimicrobial, anti-inflammatory, angiogenic, and proliferative and remodeling activity. In an effort to evaluate the antimicrobial function, an in vitro study by Mao and colleagues[37] found that human cryopreserved viable placental tissues released soluble antimicrobial peptides, including defensins and secretory leukocyte protease inhibitor, which mediate biofilm (particularly that of *Pseudomonas aeruginosa* and *Staphylococcus aureus*) formation, with the quantities of those factors differing between amnion and umbilical tissue products. As biofilms pose a significant roadblock with the release of inflammatory cytokines, further perpetuating the inflammatory phase, this could be a critical modulatory function of amnion products.[38]

Koob and colleagues[20] have been exceptionally prolific in reporting on the different mechanisms of action of amnion and chorion products. In 1 early study, they demonstrated that dehydrated human amnion and chorion membrane contain chemokines and cytokines that directly stimulate lymphocytes, affecting the inflammatory cascade. These factors that are thought to modulate inflammation and play a role in cell proliferation and tissue remodeling, which is critical for wounds stalled in the inflammatory phase of healing.[39,40]

Interestingly, this group also reported that dHACM induced proliferation of fibroblasts in vitro, and found that dHACM-treated fibroblasts upregulated growth factors known to play a role in wound healing. They also reported that dHACM induced proliferation of fibroblasts.[20] A few of these key, upregulated growth factors brought to the wound environment include epidermal growth factor (EGF), basic fibroblast growth factor (bFGF), transforming growth factors (TGF) alpha and beta, and nerve growth factor (NGF).[40]

In regards to the quantity of factors contributed by these products, it has been established that the chorion is approximately 5 times the size of the amnion layer, and is consequently 5 times more effective at inducing cell proliferation. The Koob group additionally examined the individual cytokines and growth factors provided by each layer, and found that although amnion contributes a higher percentage of

EGF, the chorion layer contributes higher percentages of PDGF-AA and VEGF.[40] They also demonstrated that angiogenic cytokines in dHACM promoted human microvascular endothelial cell proliferation in vitro. Additionally, subcutaneous dHACM implants in murine in vivo models showed an increase in the formation of new blood vessels.[41] This work provides novel insight into the angiogenic potential of these products, further explaining the mechanisms behind their unique therapeutic capacity. A thorough understanding of the factors present in amniotic tissue and their individual effects will ultimately provide a mechanism in overcoming the stagnation of wound healing and promoting tissue regeneration.

CLINICAL EVIDENCE SUPPORTING AMNIOTIC TISSUE IN WOUND CARE

A greater body of evidence exists for combined bilayer amnion and chorion products, rather than for amnion products alone. Regrettably, there are no studies directly comparing the efficacy of amnion products with that of bilayer amnion chorion allografts for wound healing, presenting a valuable area of study for future research endeavors.

A recent review and meta-analysis by Laurent and colleagues[42] looked at the combined data among 5 landmark amnion product studies. They concluded that human amnion/chorion membrane products in addition to standard of care wound care (SOC) healed diabetic foot ulcers (DFUs) significantly faster than SOC alone. Of note, this review also confirmed that ideal time points to measure healing were at 4 and 12 weeks. Another review indirectly compared 9 different dressing methodologies based on all available randomized trials, based on 17 single-center trials and 4 multi-center trials. The rank probabilities from being the most effective to least effective treatment were as follows: amniotic membrane, hydrogel, silver-impregnated, foam, honey-impregnated, alginate, basic, hydrocolloid, and iodine-impregnated dressings. Although 1 study did have a sponsor bias, this head-to-head comparison demonstrated that amniotic membrane dressings were significantly superior to others in healing DFUs[43] (**Figs. 2** and **3**).

In regards to amnion products alone, a milestone randomized controlled trial by Lavery and colleagues[44] studied the effects of a cryopreserved amnion product on DFUs present for at least 4 weeks. This study showed that when the cryopreserved amnion product was added to SOC, 62% of patients achieved healing, compared with 21.3% of those receiving SOC therapy alone. Moreover, of these healed patients, the cryopreserved amnion group demonstrated higher rates of remaining healed (82.1% vs 70%) within a 12-week follow-up period. This group's findings strongly support the addition of amnion products to promote repeat epithelialization for wounds that have stagnated in the healing process.

Tettelbach and colleagues[45] published a randomized, multicenter clinical trial throughout 14 US wound care centers examining the efficacy of dehydrated human amnion/chorion membrane (dHACM) for chronic lower extremity wounds (duration >4 weeks) in the diabetic population. Patients with less than or equal to 25% wound closure after 2 weeks of standard first-line treatment with traditional offloading and wound care were included (n = 110). One group was randomly assigned to receive weekly dHACM applications (n = 54). The allograft-treated patients demonstrated significantly reduced time to healing, being twice as likely to heal within 12 weeks compared with the group that did not receive allograft treatment. Interestingly, the allograft group demonstrated that 95% of healed ulcers remained closed at 16-week follow-up, as opposed to 86% remaining closed in the non-dHACM group. This study is among the larger studies demonstrating that dHACM products have a

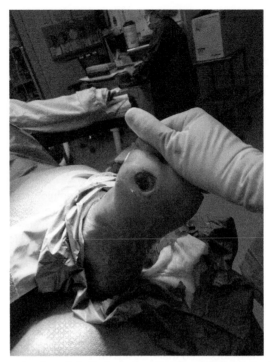

Fig. 2. A chronic, nonhealing diabetic foot ulcer that has failed standard therapy.

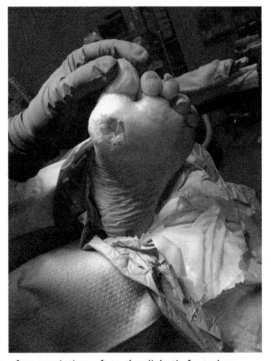

Fig. 3. Application of an amniotic graft to the diabetic foot ulcer.

significant impact on reduced time to healing, as well as continued healing for diabetic foot ulcerations.

DiDomenico and colleagues[46] also studied the use of bilayer amnion and chorion allograft in chronic foot ulcers. This randomized controlled trial was similarly designed, including 80 patients who had failed standard of care wound treatment for 2 weeks, allocating half the patients to receive dehydrated human amnion and chorion allograft treatment (dHACA). They found that at 12 weeks, 85% (34/40) of the patients treated with dHACA had healed, compared with 33% (13/40) of those treated with SOC wound care alone, with mean time to heal being significantly faster for the treated group compared with the SOC group (37 days vs 67 days, respectively).

A unique study published by the Zelen group in 2015 compared the clinical outcomes of patients with chronic lower extremity diabetic ulcers treated with bioengineered skin substitute, dHACM, and standard wound care.[47] This study included type 1 and type 2 diabetics, and randomized patients in a 1:1:1 ratio between the 3 groups. Within the 12-week study, the percentage of wounds that went on to complete closure were 73% (24/33) in the bioengineered skin substitute group, 97% (31/32) in the dHACM group, and 51% (18/35) in the standard wound care group. This is the only study to date to compare these 2 novel types of wound care products against standard therapy that demonstrated improved wound healing rates in the dHACM-treated group.

Although the bulk of data on amnion products and wound healing is focused on diabetic foot ulcerations, the scope of applications for amnion products is being widened. One recent retrospective review conducted in an outpatient podiatric surgery clinic looked at patients with wounds of various etiologies being treated with dHACM allografts.[48] All patients in both surgical (n = 21) and traumatic (n = 2) wound groups achieved complete healing. Interestingly, patients in neuropathic, venous stasis, and pressure ulcer groups achieved greater than 90% rates of healing. Of note, the only wounds that did not respond to dHACM treatment were ischemic ulcers. This study provides unique insight into a broader set of possible applications for amnion products, and should stimulate questions about if and how these products could be applied in the setting of vascular compromise.

Chronic wounds are not the only area for potential amniotic tissue applications. One novel study by Bemenderfer and colleagues[49] examined the effects of an amnion product on acute surgical wound healing after total ankle arthroplasty (TAA). A unique feature of this study was the application of amniotic membrane-umbilical cord (AM-UC) allograft at the time of primary skin closure in one group (n= 54) with no allograft application in the control group (n=50). The major finding was a decreased time to skin healing: 28.5 days in the allograft group compared with 40 days in the control group. However, both groups showed no significant difference in reoperation rate for wound complications, skin dehiscence, or need for antibiotics because of infection. Although the decreased time to healing would infer an overall decrease in skin and soft tissue complications, larger studies are likely needed to further study the effects of amnion products in postsurgical wound healing.

Exclusion criteria for these studies generally include a host of complicating factors that are often present at the time of presentation. Some of these criteria include active infection at the wound site, poor glycemic control (HbA1C >12%), wounds that probe deep to tendon/capsule/bone, and patients with reduced perfusion and suspected vascular compromise to the area.[45] This list describes a large percentage of the patient population, particularly when it comes to inadequate tissue perfusion. Teasing out why these products are significantly less effective in vasculopathic patients would be of value, as their independent angiogenic potential has been touted.[46] Looking forward, further research may address the use of amnion and chorion products in the setting of infection with concomitant antibiosis and/or surgical debridement. It might also be worthwhile to examine the timing of the use of these products surrounding vascular interventions for patients with significant vascular compromise (**Fig. 4**).

COST-EFFECTIVENESS OF AMNIOTIC TISSUE

The clinical benefits of utilizing amnion products as part of a local wound care regimen for difficult to treat wounds are numerous, and are increasingly being studied. Although these products can be of enormous value in patient outcomes, some of the logistical benefits to the provider include cost and reduced waste of material. Although these products do initially present an added cost, reduced mean time to healing also has to also be considered in the cost benefit equation. The Lavery[44] group discovered that the mean time to healing with the cryopreserved amnion product was 42 days compared with 69.5 days in the control group. Similarly, the Zelen[50] study reports a 50% reduction in time to healing in the dHACM group compared with the control group. The marked decrease in time to complete healing clearly presents a savings in office visits and physician time, possible complications, and patient quality of life.

In terms of storing amnion and chorion products, Zelen and colleagues[47] compared the ease of storage of dHACM products versus a bilayered biological skin substitute. Although dHACM can be stored at room temperatures for 5 years, biological skin substitutes generally have specific storage temperature parameters with a shelf-life of approximately 14 days. In comparing the number of applications required for wound closure between dHACM and the bilayered biological skin substitute, they additionally

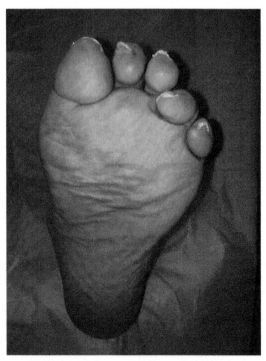

Fig. 4. Healed diabetic foot ulcer after amniotic tissue application.

reported that the dHACM group required on average 58% fewer graft applications than those receiving the bilayered biological skin substitute, with a subsequent reduction in cost. Their study reports median graft cost was $8918 (range $1486–$19,323) per healed wound for the Apligraf group and $1517 (range $434–$25,710) per healed wound in the dHACM group.

SUMMARY

Amnion and chorion products show great promise, and have real potential to be mainstays of treatment for chronic, nonhealing wounds. Although amniotic products do carry a cost, the decrease in time to healing, with the assumed subsequent decrease in complication and infection rates, should also be taken into consideration. These products, with their unique biological potential and availability in the clinical setting, may prove to be beneficial in an incredibly vast array of podiatric surgical applications.

REFERENCES

1. John T. Human amniotic membrane transplantation: past, present, and future. Ophthalmol Clin North Am 2003;16:43–65.
2. Liu J, Sheha H, Fu Y, et al. Update on amniotic membrane transplantation. Expert Rev Ophthalmol 2010;5:645–61.
3. Díaz-Prado S, Muiños-Lopez E, Hermida-Gómez T, et al. Human amniotic membrane as an alternative source of stem cells for regenerative medicine. Differentiation 2011;81(3):162–71.
4. Subrahmanyam M. Amniotic membrane as a cover for microskin grafts. Br J Plast Surg 1995;48(7):477–8.
5. Sakuragawa N, Kakinuma K, Kikuchi A, et al. Human amnion mesenchyme cells express phenotypes of neuroglial progenitor cells. J Neurosci Res 2004;78(2): 208–14.
6. Serena TE, Carter MJ, Le LT, et al. EpiFix VLUSG. A multicenter, randomized, controlled clinical trial evaluating the use of dehydrated human amnion/chorion membrane allografts and multilayer compression therapy vs. multilayer compression therapy alone in the treatment of venous leg ulcers. Wound Repair Regen 2014;22:688–93.
7. Zelen CM, Poka A, Andrews J. Prospective, randomized, blinded, comparative study of injectable micronized dehydrated amniotic/chorionic membrane allograft for plantar fasciitis—a feasibility study. Foot Ankle Int 2013;34:1332–9.
8. Adinolfi M, Akle CA, McColl I, et al. Expression of HLA antigens, beta 2-microglobulin and enzymes by human amniotic epithelial cells. Nature 1982;295(5847): 325–7.
9. Lo DD, Zimmermann AS, Nauta A, et al. Scarless fetal skin wound healing update. Birth Defects Res C Embryo Today 2012;96:237–47.
10. Leung A, Crombleholme TM, Keswani SG. Fetal wound healing: implications for minimal scar formation. Curr Opin Pediatr 2012;24:371–8.
11. Hao Y, Ma DH, Hwang DG, et al. Identification of antiangiogenic and antiinflammatory proteins in human amniotic membrane. Cornea 2000;19:348–52.
12. Liechty KW, Adzick NS, Crombleholme TM. Diminished interleukin 6 (IL-6) production during scarless human fetal wound repair. Cytokine 2000;12:671–6.
13. Tseng SC, Li DQ, Ma X. Suppression of transforming growth factor-beta isoforms, TGF-beta receptor type II, and myofibroblast differentiation in cultured human corneal and limbal fibroblasts by amniotic membrane matrix. J Cell Physiol 1999;179:325–35.

14. Penn JW, Grobbelaar AO, Rolfe KJ. The role of the TGF-beta family in wound healing, burns, and scarring: a review. Int J Burns Trauma 2012;2:18–28.
15. Lee SB, Li DQ, Tan DT, et al. Suppression of TGF-beta signaling in both normal conjunctival fibroblasts and pterygial body fibroblasts by amniotic membrane. Curr Eye Res 2000;20:325–34.
16. Lin RY, Adzik NS. The role of the fetal fibroblast and transforming growth factor-beta in a model of human fetal wound repair. Semin Pediatr Surg 1996;5:165–74.
17. Longaker MT, Adzick NS, Hall JL, et al. Studies in fetal wound healing, VII. Fetal wound healing may be modulated by hyaluronic acid stimulating activity in amniotic fluid. J Pediatr Surg 1990;25(4):430–3.
18. Zgheib J, Xu J, Liechty KW. Targeting inflammatory cytokines and extracellular matrix composition to promote wound regeneration. Adv Wound Care (New Rochelle) 2014;3:344–55.
19. Nonaka T, Kikuchi H, Ikeda T, et al. Hyaluronic acid inhibits the expression of u-PA, PAI-1, and u-PAR in human synovial fibroblasts of osteoarthritis and rheumatoid arthritis. J Rheumatol 2000;27:997–1004.
20. Koob TJ, Lim JJ, Massee M, et al. Properties of dehydrated human amnion/chorion composite grafts: implications for wound repair and soft tissue regeneration. J Biomed Mater Res B Appl Biomater 2014;102:1353–62.
21. Niknejad H, Deihim T, Solati-Hashjin M, et al. The effects of preservation procedures on amniotic membrane's ability to serve as a substrate for cultivation of endothelial cells. Cryobiology 2011;63:145–51.
22. Philip J, Hackl F, Canseco JA, et al. Amnion-derived multipotent progenitor cells improve Achilles tendon repair in rats. Eplasty 2013;13:e31.
23. Demirkan F, Colakoglu N, Herek O, et al. The use of amniotic membrane in flexor tendon repair: an experimental model. Arch Orthop Trauma Surg 2002;122(07):396–9.
24. Anderson J, Swayzee Z. The use of human amniotic allograft on osteochondritis dissecans of the talar dome: a comparison with and without allografts in arthroscopically treated ankles. Surg Sci 2015;06:412–7.
25. Riddle DL, Schappert SM. Volume of ambulatory care visits and patterns of care for patients diagnosed with plantar fasciitis: a national study of medical doctors. Foot Ankle Int 2004;25(5):303–10.
26. Goldin M, Malanga GA. Tendinopathy: a review of the pathophysiology and evidence for treatment. Phys Sportsmed 2013;41(3):36–49.
27. Andres BM, Murrell GAC. Treatment of tendinopathy: what works, what does not, and what is on the horizon. Clin Orthop Relat Res 2008;466(7):1539–54.
28. Hanselman AE, Tidwell JE, Santrock RD. Cryopreserved human amniotic membrane injection for plantar fasciitis: a randomized, controlled, double-blind pilot study. Foot Ankle Int 2015;36(2):151–8.
29. Cazzell S, Stewart J, Agnew PS, et al. Randomized controlled trial of micronized dehydrated human amnion/chorion membrane (dHACM) injection compared to placebo for the treatment of plantar fasciitis. Foot Ankle Int 2018;39(10):1151–61.
30. Barboni B, Russo V, Curini V, et al. Achilles tendon regeneration can be improved by amniotic epithelial cell allotransplantation. Cell Transplant 2012;21:2377–95.
31. Ozgenel GY, Samli B, Ozcan M. Effects of human amniotic fluid on peritendinous adhesion formation and tendon healing after flexor tendon surgery in rabbits. J Hand Surg Am 2001;26:332–9.
32. Liu Y, Peng Y, Fang Y, et al. No midterm advantages in the middle term using small intestinal submucosa and human amniotic membrane in Achilles tendon transverse tenotomy. J Orthop Surg Res 2016;11:125.

33. Coban I, Satoglu IS, Gultekin A, et al. Effects of human amniotic fluid and membrane in the treatment of Achilles tendon ruptures in locally corticosteroid-induced Achilles tendinosis: an experimental study on rats. Foot Ankle Surg 2009;15:22–7.

34. Nussbaum SR, Carter MJ, Fife CE, et al. An economic evaluation of the impact, cost, and Medicare policy implications of chronic nonhealing wounds. Value Health 2018;21(1):27–32.

35. Steed DL, Attinger C, Colaizzi T, et al. Guidelines for the treatment of diabetic ulcers. Wound Repair Regen 2006;14(6):680–92.

36. Albert S. Cost-effective management of recalcitrant diabetic foot ulcers. Clin Podiatr Med Surg 2002;19(4):483–91.

37. Mao Y, Singh-Varma A, Hoffman T, et al. The effect of cryopreserved human placental tissues on biofilm formation of wound-associated pathogens. J Funct Biomater 2018;9(1) [pii:E3].

38. Attinger C, Wolcott R. Clinically addressing biofilm in chronic wounds. Adv Wound Care (New Rochelle) 2012;1(3):127–32.

39. Koob TJ, Rennert R, Zabek N, et al. Biological properties of dehydrated human amnion/chorion composite graft: implications for chronic wound healing. Int Wound J 2013;10(5):493–500.

40. Koob TJ, Lim JJ, Zabek N, et al. Cytokines in single layer amnion allografts compared to multilayer amnion/chorion allografts for wound healing. J Biomed Mater Res B Appl Biomater 2015;103(5):1133–40.

41. Koob TJ, Lim JJ, Massee M, et al. Angiogenic properties of dehydrated human amnion/chorion allografts: therapeutic potential for soft tissue repair and regeneration. Vasc Cell 2014;6:10.

42. Laurent I, Astere M, Wang KR, et al. Efficacy and time sensitivity of amniotic membrane treatment in patients with diabetic foot ulcers: a systematic review and meta-analysis. Diabetes Ther 2017;8(5):967–79.

43. Zhang X, Sun D, Jiang GC. Comparative efficacy of nine different dressings in healing diabetic foot ulcer: a Bayesian network analysis. J Diabetes 2018; 11(6):418–26.

44. Lavery LA, Fulmer J, Shebetka KA, et al. The efficacy and safety of Grafix((R)) for the treatment of chronic diabetic foot ulcers: results of a multi-centre, controlled, randomised, blinded, clinical trial. Int Wound J 2014;11(5):554–60.

45. Tettelbach W, Cazzell S, Reyzelman AM, et al. A confirmatory study on the efficacy of dehydrated human amnion/chorion membrane dHACM allograft in the management of diabetic foot ulcers: a prospective, multicentre, randomised, controlled study of 110 patients from 14 wound clinics. Int Wound J 2019; 16(1):19–29.

46. DiDomenico LA, Orgill DP, Galiano RD, et al. Use of an aseptically processed, dehydrated human amnion and chorion membrane improves likelihood and rate of healing in chronic diabetic foot ulcers: a prospective, randomised, multi-centre clinical trial in 80 patients. Int Wound J 2018;15(6):950–7.

47. Zelen CM, Serena TE, Gould L, et al. Treatment of chronic diabetic lower extremity ulcers with advanced therapies: a prospective, randomised, controlled, multi-centre comparative study examining clinical efficacy and cost. Int Wound J 2016; 13(2):272–82.

48. Garoufalis M, Nagesh D, Sanchez PJ, et al. Use of dehydrated human amnion/chorion membrane allografts in more than 100 patients with six major types of refractory nonhealing wounds. J Am Podiatr Med Assoc 2018;108(2):84–9.

49. Bemenderfer TB, Anderson RB, Odum SM, et al. Effects of cryopreserved amniotic membrane-umbilical cord allograft on total ankle arthroplasty wound healing. J Foot Ankle Surg 2019;58(1):97–102.
50. Zelen CM, Serena TE, Denoziere G, et al. A prospective randomised comparative parallel study of amniotic membrane wound graft in the management of diabetic foot ulcers. Int Wound J 2013;10(5):502–7.

First Metatarsophalangeal Joint Implant Options

Michelle L. Butterworth, DPM[a],*, Maria Ugrinich, DPM[b]

KEYWORDS

- MTPJ • Implants • Joint implant

KEY POINTS

- Evidence-based medicine continues to guide our treatment of patients.
- Owing to the unique characteristics of the 1st MTPJ, with its small surface area and the significant amount of multiplanar force that affects it, finding the perfect implant to allow motion and alleviate pain is still the ultimate goal.
- Although some of the older silastic and other implants may still be providing pain relief and function to patients, most have failed and caused significant bone loss along the way.
- The HemiCap implants have shown some promise in select patients and may still be a viable option in patients desiring maintenance of 1st MTPJ motion.

Hallux rigidus is a common pathologic condition of the foot affecting approximately 10% of adults.[1] It is defined by end-stage arthritis of the first metatarsophalangeal joint (1st MTPJ) with limited motion of the big toe joint in the sagittal plane. Patients mostly complain of stiffness and tenderness especially with dorsiflexion of the joint in the toe-off phase of gait or with shoes that are too narrow in the toe box. As the joint undergoes degenerative changes of the bony anatomy and cartilage as a result of trauma and the stress of ambulation, osteophytic spurring occurs along with wearing away of the cartilage. The mean age of symptoms to occur is 43 years old, and the average surgical intervention occurs at 50 years of age.[2] The condition seems to be more prevalent and symptomatic in women.[2] Unilateral presentation of symptoms of hallux rigidus occurs most often in cases of trauma, whereas 95% of cases are bilateral.[2] Radiographs are useful in the evaluation of the joint space and dorsal spurring, and an MRI can further evaluate the integrity of the cartilage and the quality of the bone and identify the presence of cysts and bone marrow edema.

Treating this condition with conservative measures including physical therapy that concentrates on intrinsic strengthening, reduction of scar tissue, and

Disclosure: The authors have nothing to disclose.
[a] Williamsburg Regional Hospital, 500 Thurgood Marshall Hwy, Suite B, Kingstree, SC 29556, USA; [b] Penn Presbyterian Medical Center, 1317 Lombard Street, Philadelphia, PA 19147, USA
* Corresponding author.
E-mail address: mbutter@ftc.net

inflammation of the joint, as well as gait training, is successful for many patients. Patients with severe hallux rigidus may derive benefit from carbon graphite turf toe plates and shoe modifications. Corticosteroid injections into the joint and along areas of inflammation can also help to relieve pain. However, when those conservative efforts fail to provide pain relief and the symptoms affect daily function and quality of life, surgical interventions are indicated. The gold standard for treatment of end-stage arthritis of the 1st MTPJ has been a 1st MTPJ arthrodesis.[3] However, stopping the motion of the joint is not in line with the goals of surgery for some patients who desire to retain joint mobility. Implant arthroplasty can provide patients with motion, more stability with gait, and propulsive power. Recent meta-analysis comparing arthrodesis of the 1st MTPJ with implant arthroplasty showed that there was no significant difference in the American Orthopaedic Foot and Ankle Society (AOFAS) hallux metatarsophalangeal interphalangeal score, patient satisfaction, reoperation rates, or complications rates between the procedures.[4] However, the visual analog scale (VAS) pain score was significantly lower for arthrodesis. The analysis of the 7 studies that qualified for the meta-analysis has shown that there is evidence for use of implants in patients who want range of motion to be kept intact.[4]

Structural changes to the 1st MTPJ may occur because of foot morphology, familial genetics, trauma, and gait. In multiple studies, the 1st MTPJ was second to the knee in the incidence and severity of degenerative morphological change (DMC).[5,6] On patient evaluation and examination, pain is most commonly noted with palpation of the spurs on the dorsal first metatarsal head and/or the proximal phalanx, and with reduction in motion secondary to cartilage thinning and erosion. Curiously, the DMC is found mostly on the plantar aspect of the metatarsal head along the sesamoids. In the specimens evaluated, the change always involved the crista, and the medial facet more so than the lateral. Interestingly, when surgical intervention of the 1st MTPJ occurs, the plantar aspect of the first metatarsal head is rarely visualized other than when the metatarsal elevator is used to loosen adhesions of the joint.

ARTHROPLASTY IMPLANT OPTIONS

1st MTPJ implants have been an alternative form for treatment of end-stage arthritis of the big toe joint for 60 years. Although 1st MTPJ arthrodesis has remained the gold standard of treatment of hallux rigidus,[7,8] fusion of the joint is not ideal to meet surgical goals for all patients. Most patients want to have functional motion in the joint, stability, and maintain length of the first ray. The concept that there will be absolutely no motion within the big toe joint after surgery is difficult for some patients to process, even though the diseased joint has not moved in decades and has developed compensatory mechanisms within the lower extremity during gait.

The goal of the 1st MTPJ implant arthroplasty procedure has been to develop an implant that is as predictable and reliable as the knee or hip joint replacements. However, it has been difficult to replicate the structural and functional aspects of the 1st MTPJ. The ideal implant should relieve pain, restore motion, improve function, maintain joint stability, restore weight bearing to the hallux, and be durable. Implants have gone through many constructs and many different materials through the years trying to achieve these goals. These constructs have included silicone spacers, single-stemmed and double-stemmed, unipolar constructs with hemi-implants for the base of the proximal phalanx of the hallux, and hemi-caps for the first metatarsal head, and bipolar constructs consisting of total joint replacements.[9] The materials have changed with technological advances, from initial use of acrylic methacrylate with bone cement to silicone single-stemmed and double-stemmed implants to the use of metal and metal alloys. With regard to implant choice selection for a patient, it is important to evaluate the articular surface of the head of the metatarsal and the base of the proximal phalanx to assess the extent of the destruction. The literature does not support one implant over another, and, most of the time, it is the surgeon's expertise and familiarity with an implant that guides the selection of hardware used for a surgery.

Complications that can arise from implant arthroplasty include silicone-induced synovitis,[10] loosening of the implant, soft tissue reactions leading to severe edema, implant fracture or destruction of the bone,[11] implant subsidence, and implant deterioration resulting in lymphadenopathy.[12] If a failed implant is to be converted to an arthrodesis, resection to a level of healthy, bleeding, viable bone is necessary for a successful fusion. If the implant failed because of mechanics or infection, there could be significant bone loss on its removal necessitating a bone graft with the fusion.

Silicone Implant Arthroplasty

Noncemented metal implants were some of the first used in the 1st MTPJ in the 1950s.[13] Owing to significant complications, including bone resorption, loosening of the implant, and instability of the implant, silicone implants soon became the material of choice. Swanson first developed 2 types of silicone hemi-interpositional implants. The first was a first metatarsal head implant, which was quickly replaced by the hallucal proximal phalangeal base implant. Swanson believed that the implant placed on this nonweight-bearing side of the joint would be more stable because it would not be subjected to excessive loading. The silicone double–stem-hinged implant then became available in the 1970s, with Swanson recommending them over the hemi-implants in cases with more significant arthrosis (**Fig. 1**). Swanson identified nonfixation of the silicone implant stems as an advantage because slight flexion reduced stress on the hinge.[14]

There were many modifications to these silicone implants through the years, including Dacron jackets to aid in fibrous tissue ingrowth for stabilization of the implant, and metal grommets to provide a protective interface between the bone and implant hinge to try to prevent breakdown of the device (**Fig. 2**). In the 1980s, dentritic synovitis became an overt clinical problem with these silicone implants, and new biomaterials were investigated, including metals and metal alloys. It is also important to note that silicone implantation is actually an *interpositional arthroplasty*, not a joint replacement procedure. The implants can help maintain the length of the toe and act as a spacer, but these implants are prone to degradation over time and, when they fail, shortening of the first ray and cock-up deformity of the hallux can result, requiring removal, replacement, or arthrodesis (**Fig. 3**).

Hemi-Implants

Hemi-implants are partial joint replacements, in which an implant is placed on 1 side of the joint. The benefit to this procedure is that there is less morbidity to the joint. These hemi-implants can either replace the proximal phalangeal base of the hallux or the first metatarsal head. Initially, hemi-implants on the proximal phalanx were used, and were favored (**Fig. 4**). It was thought that these devices would act as a spacer, maintaining

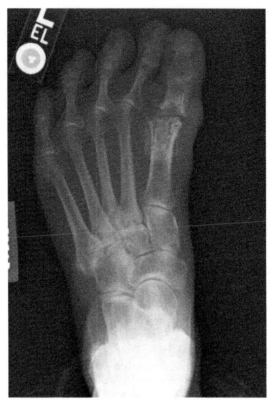

Fig. 1. Radiograph of a double-stemmed silastic implant that was placed 35 years previously. Although there is degradation of the implant the patient is still satisfied and without complaint of pain.

the length of the toe and trying to prevent recurrent breakdown of the joint following procedures such as a Keller arthroplasty or cheilectomy. They are also placed on the less weight-bearing side of the joint and therefore, are under less stress and less prone to failure.

Although phalangeal hemi-implants have been successful in decreasing pain and improving joint motion, they did not address the main anatomic location of the degeneration of the 1st MTPJ, the first metatarsal head. In the search to try to find the ideal implant, especially in younger, more active patients, resurfacing procedures of the first metatarsal head became popular and are the mainstay of joint implantation. This procedure is aimed at restoring the articular surface on the first metatarsal head. Technically, less bone is removed with resurfacing, allowing for additional options for reconstruction if future surgery is warranted secondary to implant failure.

Several first metatarsal capping devices have been developed (**Fig. 5**). Extensive research was performed on the first-generation HemiCap (Arthrosurface, Franklin, MA, USA) that was introduced on the market more than 10 years ago. It is a 2-part implant with a cobolt-chromium (CoCr) articular component and a titanium (Ti) Morse taper post for fixation into the metatarsal head. The articular aspect of the implant is contoured and cap-like, with CoCr on the articulating surface. The fixation component

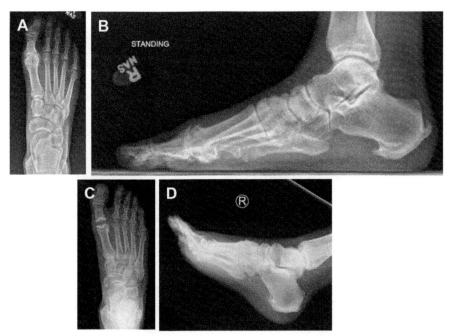

Fig. 2. (A, B) Dorsal plantar (DP) and lateral preoperative radiographs of a patient with hallux limitus and degenerative changes to the 1st MTPJ desiring implant arthroplasty. (C, D) A double-stemmed silastic implant was placed and grommets were used to increase stability and decrease the risk of degradation of the implant.

is a cannulated and tapered Ti screw for fixation into the metatarsal head. Implant insertion requires minimal bone resection of the joint and does not destabilize the intrinsic muscular insertion into the proximal phalanx[15] (**Fig. 6**). Contraindications for the HemiCap procedure include significant bone demineralization or inadequate bone stock, neuropathic changes to the foot, metal allergy or sensitivity, or history of previous osteomyelitis.[16]

A 10-year follow-up study of hemiarthroplasty patients with the HemiCap noted excellent pain relief, high patient satisfaction, low reoperation rate, and no serious complications. In addition, there was no significant change in the AOFAS scale score of 89.97 ± 8.13 from the midterm follow-up to the 10-year evaluation.[17] Other studies of 1st MTPJ arthroplasty with the HemiCap showed mean AOFAS scores of 82.1 at an average follow-up of 20 months,[18] and another study noted a mean follow-up of 37 months, with a postoperative AOFAS score of 85.1.[19] Although implant failure has been reported to be very low for the HemiCap, if it fails, surgical options can be either a Keller resection arthroplasty or a 1st MTPJ arthrodesis.[18] Because only subchondral bone is resected for the implantation of the HemiCap, there is viable bone stock for future options, with possible use of a bone graft for fusion if needed[20] (**Fig. 7**).

The most common complaint of any implant is that the dorsiflexion, which is achieved intraoperatively, is not upheld in the postoperative course. A target dorsiflexion of 90° should be achieved intraoperatively, ensuring that there are no soft tissue impingements, which will allow patients to have a postoperative range of motion that allows for smooth gait[21] (**Fig. 8**).

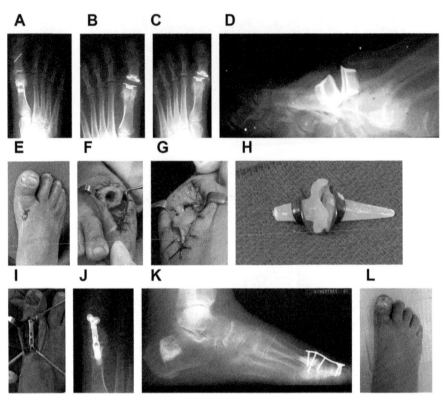

Fig. 3. (*A*) Radiograph of a patient with a distal osteotomy and Akin osteotomy to correct for a bunion deformity. (*B*) Pain persisted, and she underwent subsequent surgery with placement of a double-stemmed silicone implant with grommets. On this radiograph the implant was 10 years old. Her main complaint at this time was submetatarsal 2 pain, not 1st MTPJ pain. (*C, D*) DP and lateral radiographs 1 year after the radiograph in (*B*). Note the significant breakdown of the implant and collapse of the joint in only 1 year. The patient now has significant pain in her 1st MTPJ. (*E*) Preoperative photo of the patient. Notice the cock-up hallux secondary to failure of the implant. The patient will need removal of the implant and 1st MTPJ arthrodesis with bone graft. (*F, G*) Intraoperative photos of the first metatarsal shaft and the base of the proximal phalanx after removal of the implant and debridement. (*H*) A silastic implant that was fractured in half is realigned and grommets replaced after removal. The implant was otherwise intact except for the failure site at the hinge. (*I*) Removal of the implant and debridement back to healthy bone left a void of 1.5 cm. To maintain the length of the first ray an autogenous calcaneal bone graft was placed into the fusion site and stabilized with plate and screw fixation. (*J, K*) DP and lateral postoperative radiographs of 1st MTPJ arthrodesis with an autogenous calcaneal bone graft. (*L*) Postoperative clinical photo with good purchase of the hallux and length of the first ray maintained.

A second-generation implant for the 1st MTPJ has been developed by Arthrosurface. The current HemiCap implant used for a hemiarthroplasty of the metatarsal head has been upgraded to the HemiCap DF (Arthrosurface). The new design of the HemiCap DF has introduced a dorsal flange that is intended to improve roll-off with dorsiflexion of the 1st MTPJ in gait (**Fig. 9**). The dorsal flange DF, which curves onto the dorsal first metatarsal head, also prevents regrowth of

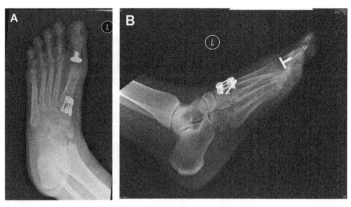

Fig. 4. (A) DP and (B) lateral radiographs of a hemi-implant on the base of the proximal phalanx of the hallux.

osteophytes, which is a common postoperative issue for hallux rigidus implant surgery (**Fig. 10**). There is a double radii of curvature built into the dorsal slope of the cap, which, at 12° of dorsiflexion of the 1st MTPJ, acts to dorsally decompress the implant. This allows the proximal phalanx to smoothly glide over the first metatarsal head[22] (**Fig. 11**). There are no studies at this time on the HemiCap DF, and all research to this point has been with the first-generation implant (**Fig. 12**).

Total Joint Replacement

During the times of increased popularity and usage of the double-stemmed silicone implants, a revolution of 2-component prostheses also occurred. The 2-component

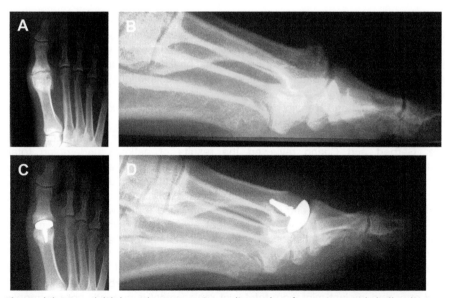

Fig. 5. (A) DP and (B) lateral preoperative radiographs of a patient with hallux limitus. Notice the decreased joint space and spurring of the first metatarsal head. (C) DP and (D) lateral postoperative radiographs after a first metatarsal head resurfacing procedure was performed with placement of a hemi-implant.

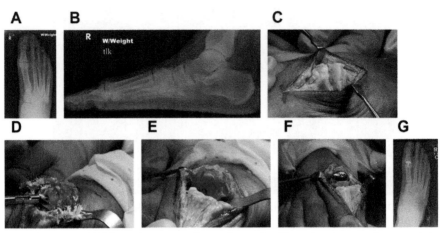

Fig. 6. (*A*) DP and (*B*) lateral preoperative radiographs. Note the decreased space of the 1st MTPJ, flattening of the first metatarsal head, and spurring of the dorsal first metatarsal head and the proximal phalanx. (*C*) Intraoperative photo showing significant degenerative changes with cartilage erosion on the first metatarsal head and spurring throughout the 1st MTPJ. (*D*) Reamer debriding the cartilage from the first metatarsal head. Placement of the guide pin should be checked with fluoroscopy before this resurfacing to ensure adequate alignment. (*E*) Fitting and evaluation of trial sizers is performed before placement of the permanent implant to ensure proper size. All bone debridement and contouring should be performed with the trial sizer in place to avoid damage to the actual implant. (*F*) Intraoperative view of the final implant placement. (*G*) Postoperative radiograph displaying good placement of the hemi-implant.

systems became favored because each component essentially functioned independently of the other (**Fig. 13**). This is a clear mechanical advantage when considering the migratory axis of the 1st MTPJ. Essential to the success of these procedures is aggressive resection of the base of the proximal phalanx to reduce tension and jamming of the joint and reattachment of the flexor hallucis longus tendon to maintain hallux purchase.

In 1996, Koenig and Horwitz[23] reported an 83.5% rate of excellent results with a 5-year follow-up using the Koenig Biomet 2-component implant. However, Boberg[18] evaluated the same population and had a much lower patient satisfaction rate. Gerbert and Chang reviewed the results of patients undergoing total joint replacement with Acumed or Bioaction implants with a 2-year follow-up. More than one-third of the patients reported complications including flexor tendonitis, metatarsalgia, sesamoid problems, metallosis, limited joint motion, and continued pain.[24] Gerbert and colleagues[25] continued to follow these patients for a 4- to 5-year follow-up, and reported that although the joint range of motion was not ideal, patient satisfaction was overall satisfactory, and their pain was minimal.

Because most of the reports on these total joint replacement systems have been inconclusive, and many of these devices have had to be removed as a result of technical error and implant migration, total joint replacement is currently not commonly used. With the advancement of technology, however, these 2-component devices have been modified and improved over time. Most of the total joint replacement systems now have a screw type of stem to provide more stability and to try to prevent

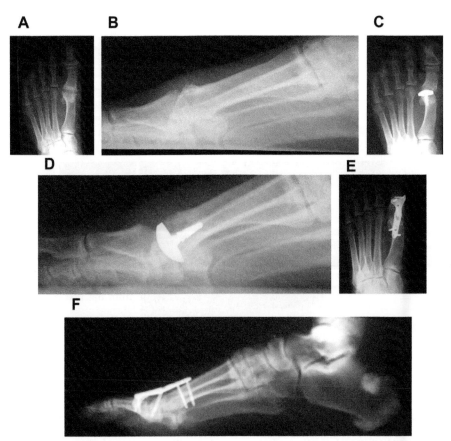

Fig. 7. (*A*) DP and (*B*) lateral radiographs of a patient who previously underwent a bunionectomy including some resection of the base the proximal phalanx. She had continued pain at the 1st MTPJ. (*C*, *D*) A first metatarsal capping procedure was performed, but her 1st MTPJ was in poor alignment and painful restricted joint motion persisted. Note the lateral angulation of the implant secondary to the positioning to the first metatarsal head and the medial deviation of the hallux. (*E*, *F*) A 1st MTPJ arthrodesis was performed and autogenous calcaneal bone graft was necessary to maintain the length of the 1st MTPJ.

migration and failure of the implant. With these newer implants, total joint replacement may still be an option in those patients who desire maintenance of 1st MTPJ motion but have extensive degeneration of the 1st MTPJ affecting both the base of the proximal phalanx of the hallux and the first metatarsal head (**Fig. 14**). Another indication for a total joint replacement includes a patient with a 1st MTPJ arthrodesis but who is dissatisfied with the results and want motion returned to their joint (**Fig. 15**).

Synthetic Cartilage Implant: Polyvinyl Alcohol Hydrogel

The novel polyvinyl alcohol (PVA) hydrogel implant (CARTIVA Synthetic Cartilage Implant; Cartiva, Inc, Alpharetta, GA, USA) received Food and Drug Administration (FDA) approval in July 2016 (**Fig. 16**). It was trialed in the United Kingdom and

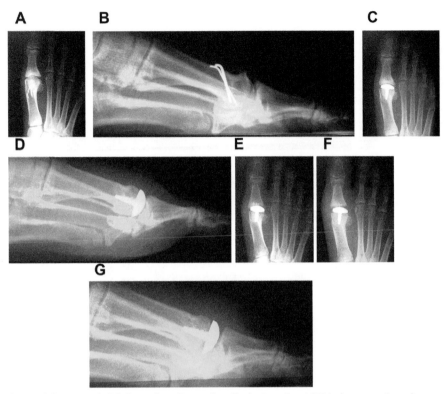

Fig. 8. (*A*) DP and (*B*) lateral radiographs displaying 1st MTPJ degenerative changes with spurring of the first metatarsal head and decreased joint space status-post (S/P) (scatter-to-primary radiation) bunionectomy several years previously. (*C, D*) Postoperative radiographs of a first metatarsal resurfacing procedure with placement of a hemi-implant. (*E*) Twelve months after the first metatarsal capping procedure was performed. Notice the decreased joint space compared with her immediate postoperative radiographs. If adequate motion is not obtained after placement of the implant, restricted motion will continue and jamming of the joint will result. (*F, G*) A resection arthroplasty was performed on the base of the proximal phalanx of the hallux. The hemi-implant was left in place. This increased joint space and range of motion of the 1st MTPJ and alleviated the pain.

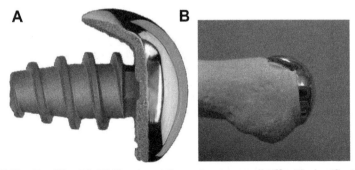

Fig. 9. (*A*) The HemiCap DF. (*B*) The dorsal flange improves roll-off with dorsiflexion of the 1st MTPJ and prevents regrowth of osteophytes. (*Courtesy of* Arthrosurface, Franklin, MA; with permission.)

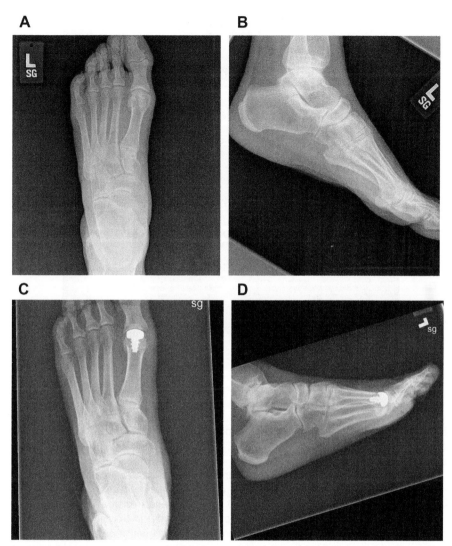

Fig. 10. (A) Preoperative DP and (B) lateral radiograph of a first metatarsal resurfacing procedure. (C, D) Placement of the HemiCap DF. The dorsal flange allows the proximal phalanx to glide smoothly over the first metatarsal head. (Arthrosurface, Franklin, MA.)

Canada and 2 studies have shown promising results before entering the United States marketplace.[26,27] The implant is made of PVA hydrogel and, when implanted, acts as a bumper or a spacer between the first metatarsal and the base of the proximal phalanx. PVA is used in contact lenses, nerve glide agents, and even food packaging because it is nontoxic and noncarcinogenic. It has no silicone, so the inflammation noted with silicone implants over time is not a concern. PVA hydrogel has properties that are similar to healthy human articular cartilage. It has a comparable ultimate tensile strength (the ability of a material to resist loads that pull it apart) with human cartilage at 17 MPa, and similar water content.[28] Initial studies in rabbits have shown that, in the immediate postoperative period,

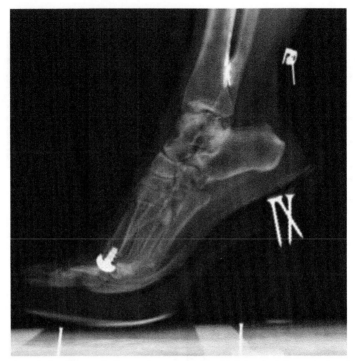

Fig. 11. Radiograph taken with the patient wearing a high-heeled shoe. Notice the amount of dorsiflexion at the 1st MTPJ and the hallux positioning on the first metatarsal head.

there is mild inflammation around the implant, which the investigators considered to be related to the surgical trauma, and, after a few weeks, the inflammatory reaction disappeared.[15]

Two trials guided FDA approval of the Cartiva implant. In a prospective, randomized multicenter study in the United Kingdom and Canada, the authors compared the safety and efficacy of the small (8 and 10 mm) synthetic hydrogel implant with the gold standard 1st MTPJ arthrodesis for the treatment of end-stage hallux rigidus. At the conclusion of the 24-month study, there were significant decreases in VAS pain scores in the implant and the fusion groups, along with equivalent functional outcomes between the 2 groups, with no signs of bone loss or implant fracture with the Cartiva. The rate of secondary surgery for the synthetic cartilage implant group was 11%, which was equivalent to the revisional rate of the 1st MTPJ arthrodesis group at 12%.[13]

The initial 24-month study was followed by a 5-year study to evaluate the PVA hydrogel implant at 3 Canadian centers. The implant was noted to have a 5.4-year survivorship of 96%.[14] In addition, patients reported significant reduction of pain on the VAS and were satisfied with the procedure. The PVA hydrogel implant maintained function and dorsiflexion (active peak dorsiflexion of 29.7°) at the 5-year mark. Radiographic comparisons did not show any implant loosening or fracture. Although 2 patients had cysts form in the proximal phalanx, neither were symptomatic.

Patient selection for every procedure is essential to its success. A 2-year, multicenter study tried to isolate those patients in whom the PVA hydrogel implant would

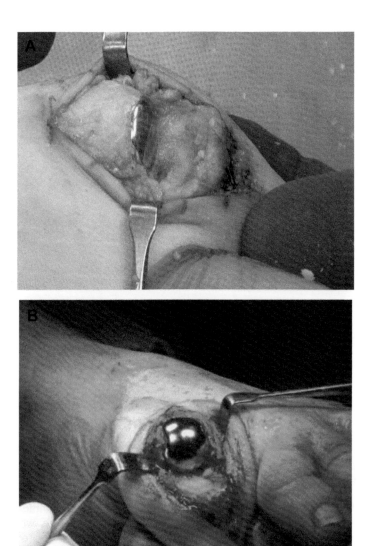

Fig. 12. Intraoperative comparison of a (A) first-generation versus (B) second-generation metatarsal hemi-implant.

be most successful. Those patients who had a pathologic condition that was classified as Coughlin grade 2, 3, or 4[29] were considered to be candidates for cartilage implants. These patients had findings of hallux rigidus with mild hallux valgus (less than or equal to 20°) and a high degree of preoperative stiffness. These findings were irrespective of sex, age, body mass index, hallux rigidus grade, preoperative pain, or duration of symptoms.[30] A more recent study has shown that, regardless of the Coughlin hallux rigidus grade, positive outcomes were noted with both arthrodesis and synthetic cartilage groups. Rather than using the Coughlin grade to decide treatment, the investigators noted that clinical symptoms and signs should guide the treatment options, because the grade could under-interpret the true extent of the arthritis in the joint.[31]

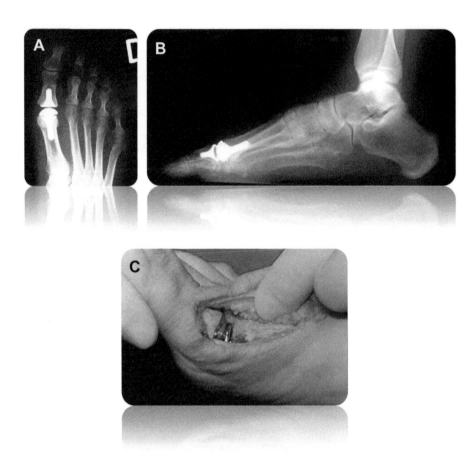

Fig. 13. (*A*) DP and (*B*) lateral radiographs showing a 1st MTPJ total joint replacement. (*C*) Intraoperative photo of the 2-component 1st MTPJ total joint replacement.

Although the aforementioned studies showed a small percentage of PVA hydrogel implant failure,[32] these results are not consistent with what United States foot and ankle surgeons are seeing. In a study recently accepted for publication, a group of surgeons performed a level IV retrospective radiographic

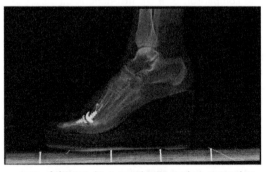

Fig. 14. The 2 components of this total joint replacement has stems that screw into the bone providing more stability. 1st MTPJ range of motion has been maintained in this patient allowing her to wear her high heels.

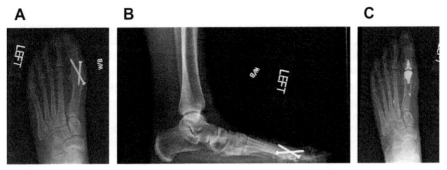

Fig. 15. (*A, B*) Radiographs of a 1st MTPJ arthrodesis and a dissatisfied patient. She has not tolerated the fusion and wants to try to regain her joint motion. Also note the abducted position of the hallux and increase in the intermetatarsal angle. (*C*) The 1st MTPJ arthrodesis was resected and a total joint replacement was performed. The 1st MTPJ must be in a rectus position for the implant to function properly, so correction of the intermetatarsal angle was obtained with a more proximal procedure.

review of 27 consecutive patients who received the implant, and measured preoperative and postoperative joint space area (JSA). A significant improvement in JSA (*P*<.001) was found between the preoperative JSA and JSA at the first post-operative visit at 1 to 2 weeks. However, a significant decrease in JSA (*P*<.001) between the first postoperative visit and the second postoperative visit at 5 to 12 weeks.[33]

The issues with the failure of these implants are multiple, as with any other failed surgery: patient pain, dissatisfaction, loss of wages, loss of quality of life, and need for further surgery. Just as bone defects are created on the removal of previous 1st MTPJ implant devices (including silastic, ceramic, and most metals), a large bone deficit is seen also with the PVA hydrogel implant. However, the bone length

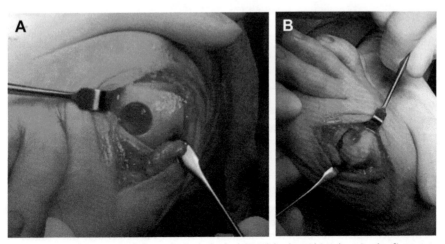

Fig. 16. (*A, B*) Placement of the polyvinyl alcohol (PVA) hydrogel implant in the first meta-tarsal head. Notice the protrusion of the implant from the first metatarsal head acting as a joint spacer.

is maintained. Traditionally, bone length loss requires *structural* autograft or allograft to restore the length of the first ray. With the Cartiva implant, the bone loss is still significant, because an intramedullary void, typically 10 mm in length and 10 mm deep, is created. Thus, bone grafting is absolutely necessary when salvaging the failure of these implants. Reactive synovitis is seen around the joint, and a biofilm develops around the implant as well and needs to be resected (**Fig. 17**).

To remove the PVA hydrogel implant, the surgical incision is the same as for insertion of the implant. The surgeon performs dissection as 1-layer to bone as in other revision surgery. Once the 1st MTPJ is exposed, allowing visualization of the metatarsal head and the proximal phalanx, the implant is evaluated, and a bone lever or osteotome is used to pry the implant from the metatarsal head and, using forceps, the implant is removed. Biopsy specimens of the tissues can be sent for culture if the surgeon prefers, but this is not essential. The metatarsal head is then denuded of cartilage to bleeding bone for arthrodesis. The 10 × 10-mm void of the central aspect of the first metatarsal head and intramedullary canal is fenestrated to create a bleeding bone recipient bed and filled with calcaneal cancellous autograft. The joint is then prepared for arthrodesis and

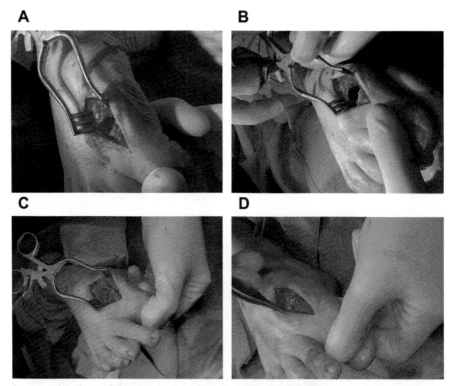

Fig. 17. (*A*) Failure of the PVA hydrogel implant. The implant appears to be flush with the first metatarsal head and is no longer maintaining adequate joint space and motion. (*B*) The PVA hydrogel implant has been removed, leaving an osseous defect that will need to be filled. (*C*) The defect in the first metatarsal is packed with autogenous calcaneal bone graft. (*D*) After packing the osseous defect with bone graft, a viable osteochondral allograft is then placed.

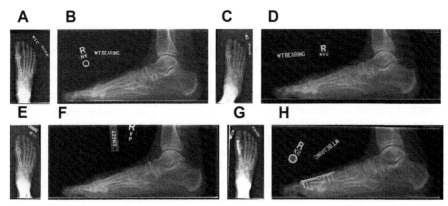

Fig. 18. (A, B) Preoperative radiographs showing degeneration of the 1st MTPJ with spurring of the first and flattening of the metatarsal head and decreased joint space. (C) DP and (D) lateral radiographs S/P 2 months after placement of a PVA hydrogel implant demonstrate maintenance of the joint space of the 1st MTPJ. (E, F) S/P 3 months after placement of the PVA hydrogel implant. Notice that, in that month, the implant has failed and the joint has collapsed. (G, H) The implant was removed and a 1st MTPJ arthrodesis was performed.

fixated with appropriate hardware. Because of bone loss, it is recommended to include an interfragmentary screw and dorsal neutralization plate, which can be eccentrically loaded to encourage compression at the arthrodesis site (**Figs. 18** and **19**). Although the concept of a hydrogel implant may seem promising, significant redesign needs to be performed to prevent subsidence of the implant and, ultimately, failure.

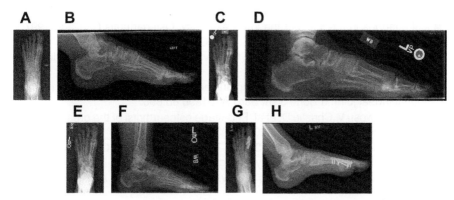

Fig. 19. (A, B) Preoperative radiographs displaying some decreased space of the 1st MTPJ and spurring of the first metatarsal head. (C, D) DP and lateral radiographs S/P 2 months after placement of a PVA hydrogel implant demonstrate maintenance of the joint space of the 1st MTPJ. (E, F) S/P 3 months after placement of the PVA hydrogel implant. The implant has failed and the joint has collapsed. (G, H) The implant was removed and a 1st MTPJ arthrodesis was performed. A large defect in the first metatarsal head required bone grafting; however, the length of the first ray was maintained; therefore, a positional graft in the 1st MTPJ is not needed.

SUMMARY

Evidence-based medicine continues to guide our treatment of patients. Because of the unique characteristics of the 1st MTPJ with its small surface area and the significant amount of multiplanar force that affects it, finding the perfect implant to allow motion and alleviate pain is still the ultimate goal. Although some of the older silastic and other implants may still be providing pain relief and function to patients, most have failed and caused significant bone loss along the way. The HemiCap implants have shown some promise in select patients and may still be a viable option in patients desiring maintenance of 1st MTPJ motion. Unfortunately, the PVA hydrogel implant has not received clinical application here in the United States, as the US FDA approval driving studies have shown. Currently, with the lack of PVA hydrogel implant studies, we do not know the true revision rates and pain scores at 10 years or more. As future research redefines optimal techniques, durability of implants and long-term functional outcomes, new advances, and next-generation products will continue to improve on the safety profile of the implants and, ultimately, patient satisfaction.

REFERENCES

1. Gould N, Schneider W, Ashikaga T. Epidemiological survey of foot problems in the continental United States: 1978-1979. Foot Ankle 1980;1:8–10.
2. Coughlin MJ, Shurnas PS. Hallux rigidus: demographics, etiology, and radiographic assessment. Foot Ankle Int 2003;24(10):731–43.
3. Lombardi CM, Silhanek AD, Connolly FG, et al. First metatarsophalangeal arthrodesis for treatment of hallux rigidus: a retrospective study. J Foot Ankle Surg 2001;40:137–43.
4. Park YH, Jung JH, Kang SH, et al. Implant arthroplasty versus arthrodesis for the treatment of advanced hallux rigidus: a meta-analysis of comparative studies. J Foot Ankle Surg 2019;58(1):137–43.
5. Heine J. Uber die arthritis deformans. Arach Path Anat Physiol 1926;260: 521–663.
6. Muehleman C, Bareither D, Huch K, et al. Prevalence of degenerative morphological changes in the joints of the lower extremity. Osteoarthritis Cartilage 1997;5: 23–37.
7. Brage ME, Ball ST. Surgical options for salvage of end stage hallux rigidus. Foot Ankle Clin 2002;7(1):49–73.
8. Shereff MJ, Baumhauer JF. Hallux rigidus and osteoarthrosis of the first metatarsophalangeal joint. J Bone Joint Surg Am 1998;80:898.
9. Perler A, Nwosu V, Christie D, et al. End-stage ostoearthritsi of the great toe/hallux rigidus. Clin Podiatr Med Surg 2013;30:351–95.
10. Vanore J, O'Keef R, Pikscher I. Silastic implant arthroplasty. Complications and their classification. J Am Podiatry Assoc 1984;74:423.
11. Yee G, Lau J. Current concepts review: hallux rigidus. Foot Ankle Int 2008;29: 637–46.
12. Lim WT, Landrum K, Weinberger B. Silicone lymaphadenitis secondary to implant degeneration. J Foot Surg 1983;22:243.
13. Swanson AB. Concepts of flexible implant design. In: Swanson AB, editor. Flexible implant resection arthroplasty in the hand and extremities. St Louis (MO): CV Mosby; 1973. p. 47–59.
14. Swanson AB, Meester WD, Swanson G, et al. Durability of silicone implants - an in vivo study. Orthop Clin North Am 1973;4:1097–112.

15. Carpenter B, Smith J, Motley T, et al. Surgical treatment of hallux rigidus using a metatarsal head resurfacing implant: mid-term follow-up. J Foot Ankle Surg 2010; 49(4):321–5.

16. Hasselman CT, Shields N. Resurfacing of the first metatarsal head in the treatment of hallux rigidus. Tech Foot Ankle Surg 2008;7:31–40.

17. Hilario H, Garret A, Motely T, et al. Ten year follow-up of metatarsal head resurfacing implants for treatment of hallux rigidus. J Foot Ankle Surg 2017;56: 1052–7.

18. Boberg JS. Koenig total toe implant arthroplasty. In: Vickers NS, editor. Reconstructive surgery of the foot and leg: update '96. Tucker (GA): Podiatry Institute; 1996. p. 136–8.

19. Aslan H, Citak M, Bas EG, et al. Early results of HemiCAP resurfacing implant. Acta Orthop Traumatol Turc 2012;46:17–21.

20. Hopson M, Stone P, Paden M. First metatarsal head osteoarticular transfer system for salvage of a failed HemiCAP implant: a case report. J Foot Ankle Surg 2009;48:483–7.

21. Kline A, Hasselman CT. Resurfacing of the metatarsal head to treat advanced hallux rigidus. Foot Ankle Clin 2015;20:451–63.

22. San Giovanni T. Arthrosrface HemiCap resurfacing. In: Weisel S, editor. Operative technicques in orthopedic surgery. 2nd edition. Lippincott Williams & Wilkins; 2016.

23. Koenig RD, Horwitz LR. The Biomet total toe system utilizing the Koenig score: a five-year review. J Foot Ankle Surg 1996;35:23–6.

24. Gerbert J, Chang TJ. Clinical experience with two-component first MPJ implants. Clin Podiatr Med Surg 1995;12:403–13.

25. Gerbert J, Chang TJ, Hall JN. A four to five year follow up of the Acumed and Bioaction implant systems in first MPJ joints: a retrospective review of 30 cases. J Foot Ankle Surg 1998.

26. Baumhauer JF, Singh D, Glazebrook M, et al. Prospective, randomized, multicentered clinical trial assessing safety and efficacy of a synthetic cartilage implant versus first metatarsophalangeal arthrodesis in advanced hallux rigidus. Foot Ankle Int 2016;37:457–69.

27. Daniels TR, Younger AS, Penner MJ, et al. Midterm outcomes of polyvinyl alcohol hydrogel hemiarthroplasty of the first metatarsophalangeal joint in advanced hallux rigidus. Foot Ankle Int 2017;38:243–7.

28. Noguchi T, Yamamuro T, Oka M, et al. Poly(vinyl alcohol) hydrogel as an artificial articular cartilage: evaluation of biocompatibility. J Appl Biomater 1991;2: 101–7.

29. Coughlin MJ, Shurnas PS. Hallux rigidus. Grading and long-term results of operative treatment. J Bone Joint Surg Am 2003;85(11):2072–88.

30. Goldberg A, Singh D, Glazebrook M, et al. Association between patient factors and outcome of synthetic cartilage implant hemiarthroplasty vs first metatarsophalangeal joint arthrodesis in advanced hallux rigidus. Foot Ankle Int 2017;38: 1199–206.

31. Baumhauer J, Signh D, Glazebrook M, et al. Correlation of the hallux rigidus grade with motion, VAS pain, intraoperative cartilage loss and treatment success for first MTP joint arthrodesis and synthetic cartilage implant. Foot Ankle Int 2017; 38(11):1175–82.

32. Davies M, Roberts V, Chadwic C, et al. Revision of synthetic cartilage implant hemiarthroplsty of the great toe to the metatarsophalangeal joint arthrodesis;

technique and indications. Tech Foot Ankle Surg 2018. https://doi.org/10.1097/BTF.0000000000000197.

33. Shi E, Todd N, Rush S, et al. First metatarsophalangeal joint space area decreases within one month after implantation of a polyvinyl alcohol hydrogel implant: a retrospective radiographic analysis. J Foot Ankle Surg, in press.

Total Ankle Replacement Options

Amber Shane, DPM[a],*, Hannah Sahli, DPM[b]

KEYWORDS

- Ankle arthritis • Total ankle replacement • Ankle arthroplasty • Joint replacement
- Fixed-bearing implants • Mobile-bearing implants

KEY POINTS

- Ankle arthroplasty is no longer experimental and has been shown to have good clinical and functional outcomes.
- Indications for total ankle replacement are vast and the patient must be considered holistically.
- Implant options are numerous and ever evolving, each with individual design pearls.
- This article discusses most used implants on the US markets.

INTRODUCTION

End-stage arthritic changes within and around the ankle joint can be a difficult pathologic condition to treat. Although arthritis in the hip or knee is typically primary osteoarthritis, a most ankle arthritis is posttraumatic.[1] However, it can take the same toll on a patient's quality of life. Patients are looking for a solution to leave them pain free, yet maintain activity and mobility. Often, we are left with 2 options: fusion or replacement. Although ankle arthrodesis has long been the "gold standard" with high fusion rates, it is not without its own complications. Ankle arthrodesis may lead to nonunion, malunion, abnormal biomechanics, decreased gait speed, increased oxygen consumption, and degeneration of adjacent joints leading to future problematic arthritis both distal and proximal to the ankle.[2,3] The idea of total joint replacement in the ankle can be very enticing to patients and surgeons alike. The concept of a pain-free ankle with maintained motion seems to be an ideal situation. Primary concerns for ankle replacement include longevity and rate of revision.

Disclosure Statement: The authors have nothing to disclose.
[a] Department of Podiatric Surgery, Advent East Podiatric Surgical Residency, Advent Health System, Orlando Foot and Ankle Clinic, 250 North Alafaya Trail Suite 115, Orlando, FL 32828, USA; [b] Department of Podiatric Surgery, Advent Health System, 250 North Alafaya Trail Suite 115, Orlando, FL 32828, USA
* Corresponding author.
E-mail address: ashane@orlandofootandankleclinic.com

HISTORY

The idea of total ankle replacement (TAR) is decades in the making. Lord and Maroote performed the first functional TAR in 1973. They implanted an inverted hip stem into the tibia and replaced the talus with a cemented acetabular cup into the calcaneus.[4,5] This initial design had a failure rate of almost 50%. The complexity of the ankle joint was appreciated because of the high failure rate. Simple hinge prosthesis would not suffice to recreate the complex mobility about the joint. Thus began the experimental phase of TAR designs. Worldwide design of the first generation of total ankle joints developed well into the 1980s, and the second generation into the early 2000s. The second generation showed substantial improvement yet had mild design flaws. Overall, most of these prostheses were removed from the market because of continued pain, high failure rate, subsidence, and need for revisions.

From the first generation of total ankle implants we learned important design qualities: to avoid including large bone resection, use of polymethylmethacrylate (PMMA) cement, and constrained implants. PMMA was associated with increased rates of osteolysis and loosening. Research also showed that large bone resection resulted in decreased bone density and strength, especially on the tibial side. Also, constrained implants were unable to dissipate rotational forces, which resulted in loosening as the main cause of failure. However, with unconstrained implants, instability occurred due to the excessive strain placed on surrounding soft tissues.[6] Because of these findings, the second generation had improved changes in design, biomaterials, and implant surfaces. The main features of the second generation included 2-component fixed-bearing systems with polyethylene bearing surfaces on components, more conservative bone cuts, and elimination of bone cement. Instead of using cement, the components were press-fit with a porous coating to allow for bony ingrowth. There were many successes with the second generation; however, many still resulted in osteolysis, subsidence, and revision. Advancements continued and led to the third and fourth generations of total ankle implants. These generations are characterized by a 3-component mobile-bearing system, many semi-constrained fixed-bearing systems, a lateral approach resurfacing option, and continued decrease in bone resection. More importantly, the new generations place a greater importance on medial and lateral ankle ligaments to retain joint stability postoperatively.[7]

Total ankle implants now are primarily divided into fixed and mobile-bearing constructs. The fixed-bearing design has 2 components that allow for stable articulation with a decreased risk of subluxation. This design is at a higher risk of loosening at the tibial component due to high shear forces at the bone-implant interface.[8] The mobile-bearing design has 3 components, this design allows for more flexible articulation with lower shear forces at the bone-implant interface. However, mobile-bearing implants are more susceptible to excessive anterior, posterior, or lateral subluxation of the polyethylene spacer, which can lead to malleolar impingement.[9] The differences in these 2 designs stem from total knee arthroplasty. In both total knee and total ankle arthroplasty, proper fit is crucial. In the ankle, proper fit allows for complete sagittal plane motion as well as axial rotation. Axial rotation is critical for even wear of the implant. Uneven wear can lead to debris and aseptic loosening, which is the leading cause of failure in TAR. Short-term results from a 2014 comparative prospective study show that fixed-bearing implants are equivalent if not slightly better than mobile-bearing implants in clinical and radiographic assessments.[10] Although earlier it was fixed-bearing implants that had unacceptable failure rates, these implants have undergone multiple changes in design and construct that have led to better patient results.

At present, implants are predominantly fixed bearing apart from 1 mobile-bearing total ankle implant approved for use in the United States.

Over the 40 years of design development there have been changes in both indications and contraindications. Traditionally, TAR was reserved for older, thin patients with low functional demand. Indications are constantly evolving for this procedure. Patient age is often an area of debate. It was previously thought that patients younger than 50 may not be suitable for TAR. However, studies are showing good clinical and functional outcomes in patients younger than 50 as well as in patients older than 70.[11–13] However, the literature is dense with data showing increased rates of revision in younger patients;[14] with advances in surgery and in implants, age is a factor that continues to vary. Patient body weight, based on body mass index (BMI), is an additional patient factor that has evolved over time. Barg and colleagues[15] found a 93% success rate among 123 TARs at a 6-year follow-up, with a mean BMI of 32.9. They did not find that a trend for obesity affected the rate of aseptic loosening. The study even found a mild decrease in BMI 2 years postoperatively. Many have shown that obesity does not increase risk of complication, infection, or implant failure. However, patients with diabetes mellitus, with an A1c greater than 7, are at increased risk for infection and implant failure.[16] When considering a patient's activity, it is important to evaluate the type of activity they hope to perform. Low-impact sports, such as walking, golfing, swimming, and cycling are great fits for TARs and would be an indication. However, if a patient is hoping to perform high-impact exercise, activity may then be a contraindication. Local patient factors should also be considered. Ipsilateral hindfoot deformity or arthrosis, as well as contralateral ankle arthrodesis, should be considered. If a patient is at risk for a pantalar arthrodesis or bilateral ankle arthrodesis this may be an indication to recommend ankle arthroplasty to spare the ankle joint.[16] In addition to hindfoot deformity, tibiotalar joint deformity should also be evaluated. Malalignment of the joint with a TAR can cause a condition called "edge-loading." This is asymmetric loading on the polyethylene component as well as the implant-bone interface. Over time, this leads to uneven wear and thus increased risk of implant loosening.[17] Patients with a varus deformity of 20° or valgus deformity of 15° can have good results with a TAR without additional osteotomies.[16] However, the indications are increased when considering patient age, BMI, activity level, and existing deformity. Some factors to consider indicating against replacement include young, very active patients, severe lower extremity malalignment, significant osteoporosis, avascular necrosis of the talus, poor soft tissue envelope, and active smoking. Although indications and relative contraindications are changing, few static contraindications exist, including; active infection, severe peripheral vascular disease, Charcot neuroarthropathy, and peripheral neuropathy. To determine if a patient is a good fit for a TAR it is most important to look beyond the ankle joint alone and consider the patient holistically. Some whole-patient factors have been shown to have a negative impact on postoperative improvement, including depression, higher American Society of Anesthesiologists (ASA) scores, current smoking, increased length of hospital stay, and previous surgical procedures. Current smoking, factors associated with increased ASA scores, and depression are factors that could be optimized before surgery for improved outcome.[18] If the patient is a good fit, there are many total ankle implants on the market. Each implant varies in design rationale, insertion, and materials.

Mobile Bearing

The only 3-part mobile-bearing implant approved for use in the US market is the *Scandinavian Total Ankle Replacement* (STAR, Stryker Orthopedics). This implant was developed by Kofoed in 1978.[19,20] Since then, many improvements have been made, and it became available in the United States for uncemented use in 2009.[21] The tibial and talar components are coated in a titanium plasma porous coating to allow for bony ingrowth. In this mobile-bearing design, the central piece can move against both tibial and talar components, which allows for motion in all 3 cardinal planes. **Fig. 1** is an image of a current STAR total implant. This implant has over 90% 10-year survivorship based on current studies.[22,23] A more recent UK study, published in 2019 by Clough and colleagues,[24] showed long-term results for the STAR implant between 1993 and 2000. The study included 200 patients with an average age of 54 years. They found 5-, 10-, and 15.8-year survival rates of 90.1%, 82.7%, and 76.1%, respectively.

Fixed Bearing

The remaining array of total ankle implants on the market are fixed-bearing, 2-component implants with a polyethylene insert that locks into the tibial component. Each company has design differences creating multiple options for the foot and ankle surgeon. The *INBONE* (1 and 2), INFINITY, and the *INVISION* are all available from Wright Medical Technologies. The INBONE was the first to be used in intramedullary referencing implantation.[16] It was cleared for use in the United States in 2005. The *INBONE II* was released not long thereafter (**Fig. 2**). This is a new and improved version of the initial design. The new system kept key design components, such as modular tibial system, thicker polyethylene bearings, and intramedullary guidance. However, it added a sulcus articulation, additional talar fixation, longer tibial trays to insure full cortical contact, and instrumentation to aid in implantation and bone removal.[25,26] The intramedullary modularity of the INBONE II (shown in **Fig. 2**) allows for increased stability within the tibial canal. This allows for greater force distribution and decreased shear at the bone-implant interface. The distribution of forces decreases the risk of osteolysis and implant loosening.[25] This implant is also suitable for revision arthroplasties because of its intramedullary design and multiple size options. At early follow-up, the INBONE II has shown promising results. Lewis and colleagues[27] reported 97% implant survival at 2 years in 56 patients and Hsu and Haddad[28] reported 100% implant survival at 2 years in 31 patients. The INFINITY is a fourth-generation TAR ideal for patients with limited deformity, and in relatively younger patients with healthy bone stock (**Fig. 3**).[29] This implant requires limited bone resection, especially on the talar side. In addition, this implant does not require the use of extensive intraoperative devices for placement. The INFINITY implant may be used with the *Prophecy* computed tomography (CT)-guided system for patient-specific implantation (**Fig. 4**). It is not uncommon to have preserved bone quality on either the talar or tibial side, but to find

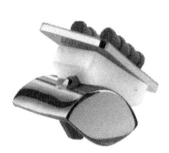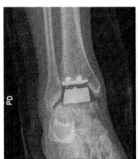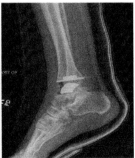

Fig. 1. Scandinavian total ankle replacement (STAR). Only mobile-bearing implant on the US Market. (*Courtesy of* Stryker, Kalamazoo, MI; with permission.)

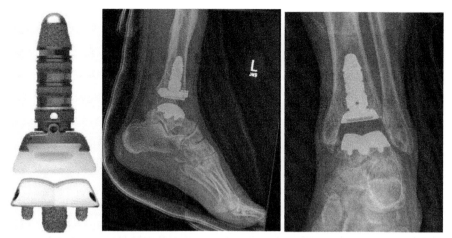

Fig. 2. INBONE II showing intramedullary modularity of the tibial component. (Image courtesy of Wright Medical Group N.V.)

poor bone stock or abundant cystic changes on the opposing side. In a patient with these findings, the INBONE II and INFINITY components may be interchanged. The *Prophecy* preoperative planning system has been shown to lead to accurate, reproducible joint alignment, decrease operative time, decrease instrumentation, increase survivorship and durability, and even decrease the learning curve in TAR.[30–32] The purpose of the system is to set the optimal position for the tibial and talar cut guides, and ultimately the implants. The key to success is a CT scan, with less than 1.25-mm slice increments, of the proximal and distal tibia, the fibula, and the talus. When the scan is ready, the surgeon receives patient-specific surface-matched operative guides with a 3D mockup of the distal tibia and the talus (as shown in **Fig. 4**). This system can be used on all Wright Medical Technologies total ankle implants. The third, and most recent, implant from Wright Medical Technologies is the INVISION. This implant was developed for revision surgeries. It is composed of a modular intramedullary tibial component and a talar plate, which comes in 2 thicknesses. This gives the ability to restore talar height.

The Salto Talaris is another fixed-bearing total ankle implant available in the United States. This implant was originally designed in the 1990s as a mobile-bearing implant

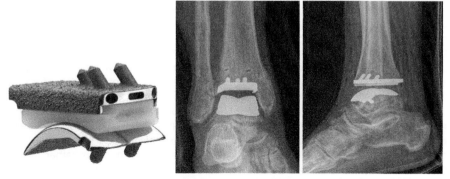

Fig. 3. INFINITY total ankle implant. (Image courtesy of Wright Medical Group N.V.)

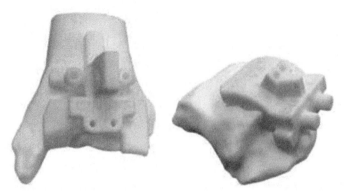

Fig. 4. Prophecy 3D mockup for preoperative planning. Allows the surgeon to visualize how the navigation guide fits on the patient's natural anatomy of the tibia and talus. This allows accurate placement of the cut guides. (Image courtesy of Wright Medical Group N.V.)

in Europe. However, after kinematic testing it was determined that, in fact, it functioned as a fixed-bearing device.[33] The fixed-bearing version was approved for use in the United States in 2006. The implant has since been redesigned multiple times optimizing the tibial plate for complete coverage. This implant also has rounded corners, both anterior medial and anterior lateral, to prevent overhang and impingement. Another interesting design feature is the biconvex talus creating a more anatomic structure. This allows for improved axial rotational alignment with the tibia. Stewart and colleagues[34] reviewed results of 106 Salto Talaris ankles at a minimum of 5-year follow-up and found a nearly 95.8% success rate. Salto Talaris also has a revision implant line: the Salto Talaris XT Revision Ankle Prosthesis. The intra-articular portions of the implant remain the same, allowing them to be interchangeable with the Salto Talaris. The tibial component has a long or short keel proximally for stable insertion and minimal bone loss. The talar component allows for flat cuts, as well as a long or short stem, again to allow for stability of the stem into healthy bone. The long stem of the talar component may be passed through the subtalar joint if additional deformity correction or arthrodesis is needed.[35]

More recent TAR implants on the market include the Cadence (Integra LifeSciences, Plainsboro, NJ) and Vantage (Exactec, Gainseville, FL) ankles. Both are fixed-bearing designs approved by the US Food and Drug Administration for use in 2016.

The Cadence has some qualities that make it stand out from the others. The polyethylene insert is made of highly crosslinked polyethylene (HXLPE), which is stronger and thus limits debris compared with the ultra-high-molecular-weight polyethylene that is used in most other implants. This HXLPE insert comes with 3 options (neutral, anterior biased, and posterior biased) allowing for correction of anterior or posterior subluxation.[36] This implant is also designed to alleviate the complication of fibular impingement with a fibular recess on the tibial component.

The Vantage total ankle is made in mobile and fixed-bearing designs; however, only the fixed-bearing design is approved for use in the United States. Following the trend in total ankle implant design, this ankle focuses on minimal bone resection and anatomic contouring (**Fig. 5**). It makes a true dome cut on the talus rather than a chamfer cut (**Fig. 6**). This implant, like the Cadence, also addresses fibular impingement with a groove cut in the tibial plate. Another distinctive design feature is its

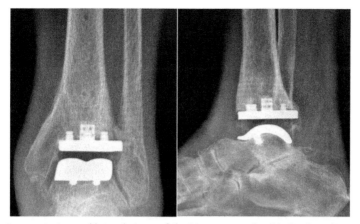

Fig. 5. Anteroposterior and lateral views of the Vantage total ankle implant (Exactech, Inc., Gainesville, FL.)

fixation. Many designs, as with this one, have pegs that insert on the tibial and talar sides. However, the Vantage also has a central vertical caged peg that inserts into the tibia for additional bony ingrowth. Who makes these?

Surgical Methods

Lateral transfibular approach
The final fixed-bearing ankle replacement to be discussed is the Trabecular Metal Total Ankle (Zimmer Biomet, Warsaw, IN) (**Fig. 7**). This implant's most distinguishing feature is the approach. The aforementioned ankles require a careful anterior ankle dissection with anterior to posterior insertion of the components. This is the only total ankle that requires a lateral approach with a fibular osteotomy. The suggested benefit of this approach is the ability to make curved bone cuts that have been shown to have a biomechanical advantage,[37] as well as a decreased risk in wound healing complications due to location. Although the anterior approach is well known for wound risks, Useulli and colleagues[38] found no significant difference in surgical

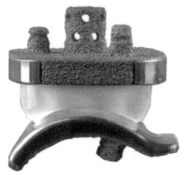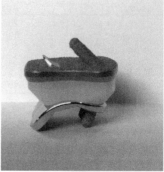

Fig. 6. The left implant is the Vantage prosthesis with true talar dome contour while the right image is an implant that shows a commonly seen chamfer cut for the talus. This image also reveals the differences in angles for tibial pegs. These are a couple of the biggest differences between fourth generation implants. (*Courtesy of* Exactech, Inc., Gainesville, FL.)

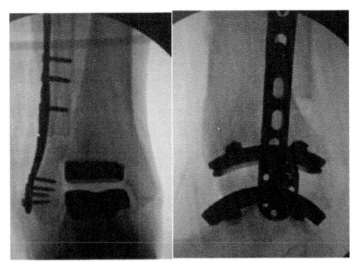

Fig. 7. AP and lateral views of the lateral approach total ankle implant.

site infection due to location. They did, however, find significant increase in surgical time in the anterior approach, because, with this lateral approach, the bone cuts on either side of the implant maintain the true contour of the ankle joint, rather than flat cuts on either side.[39] In addition to this, the medial side of the implant has a smaller radius than the lateral, which avoids stress on the collateral ligaments and allows dorsiflexion with eversion, as well as plantar flexion with inversion, to truly mimic the natural complex movements of a native ankle joint.[39] Barg and Saltzman[40] have reported 96% survival rate at 36-month follow-up with 54 patients. Usuelli and colleagues[41] had similar findings published in 2019, with 98.9% without revision or removal at 1-year follow-up.

Table 1
Review of current literature revealing survival rates of available implants in the United States

	Study	Number of Ankles	Mean Age (y)	Survival Rates 2 y	5 y	10 y	15 y
STAR	Clough et al,[24] 2019	200	54	NR	90%	83%	76%
	Loewy et al,[42] 2019	138	62	NR	90%	82%	77%
	Frigg et al,[43] 2017	50	58	NR	92%	90%	87%
	Koivu et al,[44] 2017	34	53	NR	94%	87%	64%
	Jastifer & Coughlin,[22] 2015	18	61	NR	NR	94%	NR
	Brunner et al,[45] 2013	77	57	NR	NR	71%	NR
Salto Talaris	Koo et al,[46] 2018	55	70	NR	93%	NR	NR
	Stewart et al,[34] 2017	72	62	100%	96%	NR	NR
INBONE II	Lewis et al,[27] 2015	56	60	97%	NR	NR	NR
INFINITY	Penner et al,[47] 2018	67	62	97%	NR	NR	NR
Trabecular Metal	Barg et al,[48] 2018	55	67	93%	NR	NR	NR

Implants not mentioned above that are available also include INBONE, INVISION, Vantage, and Cadence. No literature is available at this time for survival rates of the implants not included.
    Abbreviation: NR, not reported.

Total ankle arthroplasty has had significant advances in the last 50 years, and continues to evolve. With new implant designs and advancements in surgical technique, survival rates continue to improve (**Table 1**). Careful patient selection, knowledge of implant options, and thorough postoperative protocol can yield excellent clinical and functional results. Total ankle arthroplasty has proved to be a viable option for end-stage ankle arthritis. Continued research on long-term results to support longevity and durability is still needed.

REFERENCES

1. Valderrasano V, Horsserger M, Russell I, et al. Etiology of ankle osteoarthritis. Clin Orthop Relat Res 2009;467(7):1800–6.
2. Hahn ME, Wright ES, Segal AD, et al. Comparative gait analysis of ankle arthrodesis and arthroplasty: initial findings of a prospective study. Foot Ankle Int 2012; 33(4):282–9.
3. DeHeer PA, Catoire SM, Taulman J, et al. Ankle arthrodesis: a literature review. Clin Podiatr Med Surg 2012;29(4):509–27.
4. Lord G, Marotte JH. Total ankle prosthesis. Technic and 1st results. Apropos of 12 cases. Rev Chir Orthop Reparatrice Appar Mot 1973;59(2):139–51.
5. Lord G, Marotte JH. Total ankle replacement. Rev Chir Orthop Reparatrice Appar Mot 1980;66(8):527–30.
6. Bonasia DE, Dettoni F, Femino JE, et al. Total ankle replacement: why, when and how? Iowa Orthop J 2010;30:119.
7. Brandão RA, Prissel MA, Hyer CF. Current and emerging insight on total ankle replacement. Podiatry Today 2018;31:36–43.
8. Valderrabano V, Pagenstert GI, Muller AM, et al. Mobile- and fixed-bearing total ankle prostheses: is there really a difference? Foot Ankle Clin 2012;17(4):565–85.
9. Conti SF, Wong YS. Complications of total ankle replacement. Clin Orthop Relat Res 2001;391:105–14.
10. Gaudot F. A controlled, comparative study of a fixed-bearing versus mobile-bearing ankle arthroplasty. Foot Ankle Int 2014;35(2):131–40.
11. Kofoed H, Lundberg-Jensen A. Ankle arthroplasty in patients younger and older than 50 years: a prospective series with long term follow up. Foot Ankle Int 1999; 20:501–6.
12. Rodriques-Pinto R, Muras J, Martin O, et al. Total ankle replacement in patients under the age of 50. Should the indications be revised? Foot Ankle Surg 2013; 19:229–33.
13. Tenenbaum S, Bariteau J, Coleman S, et al. Functional and clinical outcomes of total ankle arthroplasty in elderly compared to younger patients. Foot Ankle Surg 2017;23:102–7.
14. Scott RT, Hyer CF, Berlet GC. Primary INBONE total ankle systems. In: Roukis TS, Berlet GC, Bibbo C, et al, editors. Primary and revision total ankle replacement; evidence- based surgical management. New York: Springer International Publishing; 2016. p. 70.
15. Barg A, Knupp M, Anderson AE, et al. Total ankle replacement in obese patients: component stability, weight change and functional outcome in 118 consecutive patients. Foot Ankle Int 2011;32:925–32.
16. Cody EA, Scott DJ, Easley ME. Total ankle arthroplasty, a critical analysis review. JBJS Rev 2018;6(8):e8.
17. Henricson A, Agren P-H. Secondary surgery after total ankle replacement, the influence of preoperative hindfoot alignment. Foot Ankle Surg 2007;13:41–4.

18. Cunningham DJ, DeOrio JK, Nunley JA, et al. The effect of patient characteristics on 1 to 2-year and minimum 5-year outcomes after total ankle arthroplasty. J Bone Joint Surg Am 2019;101(3):199–208.

19. Gougoulias N, Maffulli N. History of total ankle replacement. Clin Podiatr Med Surg 2013;30(1):1–20.

20. American Orthopedic Foot and Ankle Society. Total ankle replacement (TAR). Ortho-paedicsOne- The Orthopaedic Knowledge Network; 2009. p. 318–72. Available at: https://www.orthopaedicsone.com/pages/viewpage.action?pageId=27099870.

21. Gougoulias N, Maulli N. History of total ankle replacement in North America. In: Roukis TS, Berlet GC, Bibbo C, et al, editors. Primary and revision total ankle replacement: evidence-based surgical management. New York: Springer International Publishing; 2016. p. 3–13.

22. Jastifer JR, Coughlin MJ. Long-term follow-up of mobile bearing total ankle arthroplasty in the United States. Foot Ankle Int 2015;36(2):143–50.

23. Mann JA, Mann RA, Horton E. STAR ankle: long-term results. Foot Ankle Int 2011; 32(5):473–84.

24. Clough T, Bodo K, Majeed H, et al. Survivorship and long-term outcome of a consecutive series of 200 Scandinavian Total Ankle Replacement (STAR) implants. Bone Joint J 2019;101-B:47–54.

25. Cott RT, Hyer CF, Berlet GC. Primary INBONE total ankle systems. In: Roukis TS, Berlet GC, Bibbo C, et al, editors. Primary and revision total ankle replacement: evidence-based surgical management. New York: Springer International Publishing; 2016. p. 67–74.

26. Abicht BP, Roukis TS. The INBONE II total ankle system. Clin Podiatr Med Surg 2013;30(1):47–68.

27. Lewis JS Jr, Green CL, Adams SB Jr, et al. Comparison of first- and second-generation fixed-bearing total ankle arthroplasty using a modular intramedullary tibial component. Foot Ankle Int 2015;36(8):881–90.

28. Hsu AR, Haddad SL. Early clinical and radiographic outcomes of intramedullary-fixation total ankle arthroplasty. J Bone Joint Surg Am 2015;97(3):194–200.

29. Prissel MA, Daigre JL, Penner MJ, et al. INFINITY total ankle system. In: Roukis TS, Berlet GC, Bibbo C, et al, editors. Primary and revision total ankle replacement: evidence-based surgical management. New York: Springer International Publishing; 2016. p. 75–88.

30. Hsu AR, Davis WH, Cohen BE, et al. Radiographic outcomes of preoperative CT scan-derived patient-specific total ankle arthroplasty. Foot Ankle Int 2015;36(10): 1163–9.

31. Daigre J, Berlet G, Van Dyke B, et al. Accuracy and reproducibility using patient-specific instrumentation in total ankle arthroplasty. Foot Ankle Int 2017;38(4): 412–8.

32. Hamid KS, Matson AP, Nwachukwu BU, et al. Determining the cost-savings threshold and alignment accuracy of patient-specific instrumentation in total ankle replacements. Foot Ankle Int 2017;38(1):49–57.

33. Rush SM, Todd N. Salto Talaris fixed-bearing total ankle replacement system. Clin Podiatr Med Surg 2013;30:69–80.

34. Stewart MG, Green CL, Adams SB Jr, et al. Midterm results of the Salto Talaris total ankle arthroplasty. Foot Ankle Int 2017;38(11):1215–21.

35. Roukis TS. The Salto Talaris XT revision ankle prosthesis. Clin Podiatr Med Surg 2015;32(4):551–67.

36. Tsai J, Pedowitz DI. Next-generation, minimal-resection, fixed-bearing total ankle replacement: indications and outcomes. Clin Podiatr Med Surg 2018;35(1): 77–83.
37. Bischoff JE, Schon L, Saltzman C. Influence of geometry and depth of resections on bone support for total ankle replacement. Foot Ankle Int 2017;38(9):1026–34.
38. Usuelli FG, Indino C, Maccario C, et al. Infections in primary total ankle replacement: anterior approach versus lateral transfibular approach. Foot Ankle Surg 2019;25(1):19–23.
39. Brigido SA, DiDomenico LA. Primary Zimmer Trabecular Metal total ankle replacement. In: Roukis TS, Berlet GC, Bibbo C, et al, editors. Primary and revision total ankle replacement: evidence-based surgical management. New York: Springer International Publishing; 2016. p. 131–52.
40. Barg A, Saltzman C. Early clinical and radiographic outcomes of trabecular metal total ankle using transfibular approach: a minimum follow-up of 2 Years. AOFAS Annual Meeting. Seattle, Washington, July 12–15, 2017.
41. Usuelli FG, Maccario C, Granata F, et al. Clinical and radiological outcomes of transfibular total ankle arthroplasty. Foot Ankle Int 2019;40(1):24–33.
42. Loewy EM, Sanders TH, Walling AK. Intermediate-term experience with the STAR® total ankle in the United States. Foot Ankle Int 2019;40(3):268–75.
43. Frigg A, Germann U, Huber M, et al. Survival of the Scandinavian Total Ankle Replacement (STAR): results of ten to nineteen years follow-up. Int Orthop 2017;41(10):2075–82.
44. Koivu H, Kohonen I, Mattila K, et al. Long-term results of Scandinavian total ankle replacement. Foot Ankle Int 2017;38(7):723–31.
45. Brunner S, Barg A, Knupp M, et al. The Scandinavian Total Ankle Replacement: long-term, eleven to fifteen-year, survivorship analysis of the prosthesis in seventy-two consecutive patients. J Bone Joint Surg Am 2013;95(8):711–8.
46. Koo K, Liddle AD, Pastides PS, et al. The Salto total ankle arthroplasty—clinical and radiological outcomes at five years. Foot Ankle Surg 2018. https://doi.org/10.1016/j.fas.2018.04.003.
47. Penner M, Davis WH, Bemenderfer T, et al. The infinity total ankle system: early clinical results with 2-to 4-year follow-up. Foot Ankle Spec 2018;3(3). 2473011418S00382.
48. Barg A, Bettin CC, Burstein AH, et al. Early clinical and radiographic outcomes of trabecular metal total ankle replacement using a transfibular approach. J Bone Joint Surg Am 2018;100(6):505–15.

Orthobiologics

Tenaya A. West, DPM[a], Mitzi L. Williams, DPM[b],*

KEYWORDS

- Orthobiologics • Allograft • Autograft • Foot and ankle • Foot surgery • PRP
- Bone substitutes

KEY POINTS

- The use of orthobiologics has gained popularity in sports medicine and musculoskeletal surgery. However, clinical evidence is lacking for most commercially available and advertised products.
- The need for ongoing research to support the use of various orthobiologics is needed, especially in foot and ankle surgery.
- Although limited, the current literature supports the use of structural allografting for pediatric foot surgery. Further investigation is needed to assess safety and efficacy of other osteobiologics, specifically with osteoinductive agents.

INTRODUCTION

Orthobiologics in sports medicine and musculoskeletal surgery has garnered significant interest from physicians and patients, with increasing use over recent years.[1,2] However, many of the commercially available and advertised products lack clinical evidence.[3] The widespread use of products before fully understanding their true indications may result in unknown adverse outcomes, unfounded costs, and early failures, leading to abandonment of potentially viable treatments.[2] As more of these products become available, it is important to remain judicial in their use and to practice evidence-based medicine. Likewise, it is important to continue advances in research in the hope of improving surgical outcomes. This article reviews clinical evidence behind common orthobiologics in the treatment of foot and ankle pathology.

SOFT TISSUE

The use of orthobiologics for soft tissue injuries is prevalent in sports medicine. With athletes striving to get back to their sport, observing quick return to activity and

Disclosure: The authors have nothing to disclose.
[a] Kaiser San Francisco Bay Area Foot and Ankle Residency Program, Department of Orthopedics and Podiatric Surgery, Kaiser Foundation Hospitals, 3600 Broadway, Oakland, CA 94611, USA; [b] Kaiser San Francisco Bay Area Foot and Ankle Residency Program, Department of Orthopedics and Podiatric Surgery, 3600 Broadway, Suite 17, Oakland, CA 94611, USA
* Corresponding author.
E-mail address: mitzi.l.williams@kp.org

excellent functional results after an intervention is not unexpected. However, many orthobiologic studies lack the blinding or control groups necessary to prove that the intervention itself is effective. Platelet-rich plasma (PRP) and amniotic-derived products are 2 commonly discussed orthobiologics for accelerated rehabilitation in a multitude of acute and chronic injuries. Although the literature is still developing, there may be promise in certain applications.

Platelet-Rich Plasma

PRP is an autologous preparation of plasma with concentrated platelets, rich in growth factors, cytokines, and chemokines. Various preparations are available, most notably including leukocyte-rich PRP (LR-PRP) or leukocyte-poor PRP (LP-PRP), added anticoagulants, and exogenous activating agents.[4–6] There is widespread enthusiasm for the use of PRP products for myriad musculoskeletal applications despite conflicting evidence on their efficacy.[1]

Chronic Achilles tendinopathy

Multiple level IV noncontrolled studies have shown positive clinical results with use of PRP for chronic Achilles tendinopathy.[7] However, level I randomized controlled trials have failed to consistently show the same positive results. Improvement in Victorian Institute of Sport Assessment-Achilles (VISA-A) scores and tendon properties with use of PRP in conjunction with eccentric rehabilitation programs remains debated.[8–11] A meta-analysis of 4 randomized controlled trials failed to show a difference between PRP and saline groups in VISA-A scores, change in tendon thickness, and neovascularization, as measured by color Doppler activity.[12] Interpretation of these results is confounded by multiple PRP preparations and injection techniques, as well as the variation in activity levels, and compliance to rehabilitation regimens. It is important to consider that the injection itself, regardless of the content, may also have a beneficial effect; needling and increase in peritendinous volume have been suggested to improve symptoms in Achilles tendinopathy.[13,14]

Acute Achilles tendon ruptures

Despite strong beneficial effects of PRP augmentation in animal and immunohistochemical studies examining acute Achilles tendon ruptures,[15,16] there is, as yet, no compelling evidence to suggest improved functional outcomes *in vivo*. De Carli and colleagues[17] found no difference in patient-reported outcomes, tendon thickness, ultrasound findings, jumping capability, and return to sport when comparing 2 groups of surgically treated acute Achilles tendon ruptures, with 1 group receiving peri-operative PRP. Similarly, Kaniki and colleagues[18] showed no difference in isokinetic plantar flexion strength in conservatively treated Achilles tendon ruptures with or without PRP injections. In a comprehensive randomized, controlled trial, Schepull and colleagues[19] reported no increase in functional outcomes in Achilles tendons with repair augmented by PRP (**Figs. 1** and **2**).

There have been few studies to suggest potential functional benefit of PRP for acute Achilles tendon ruptures. In a prospective study, Zou and colleagues[20] showed increased isokinetic muscle strength at 3 months and improved patient-reported outcomes (Leppilahti scores and Short Form 36); however, the results are limited by differing surgical preparation of the tendon ends, and by a conservative rehabilitation program that did not allow for protected full weight bearing until 3 months postoperatively. Sánchez and colleagues[21] similarly looked at a group of athletes with surgically repaired acute Achilles tendon ruptures. They found a quicker return to sport in the group treated with platelet-rich fibrin matrices, compared with a retrospective matched

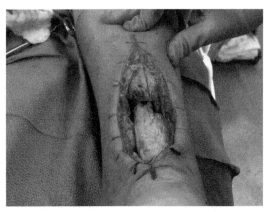

Fig. 1. Achilles tendon rupture.

surgical control group without augmentation. However, given the small sample size of 6 patients in each group, further studies must be done to validate this finding.

Ankle sprains
There are limited data available on the use of PRP in acute ankle sprains; however, interest is growing regarding use of PRP in acute syndesmotic injuries in high level athletes. A small cohort of elite athletes with complete anterior inferior tibiofibular ligament tears showed a quicker return to sport and less pain returning to activity

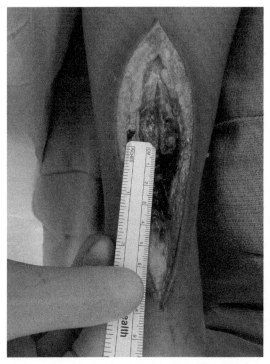

Fig. 2. Demonstrating gap distance and void of neglected Achilles tendon rupture with known history of chronic tendonosis.

when receiving ultrasound-guided PRP injections compared with those with the same rehabilitation protocol without injections (40.8 ± 8.9 vs 59.6 ± 12 days, P = .006).[22] Similarly, rugby players with syndesmotic injuries returned to sport quicker after a PRP injection compared with a retrospective cohort that had undergone the same rehabilitation protocol without PRP (48.6 ± 11.7 vs 69.3 ± 29.1 days, P = .048).[23] Of note, the athletes in both studies were not blinded to the treatment.

There is, as yet, insufficient data examining the use of PRP in lateral ankle sprains. In 2015, a small, double-blind randomized control trial examined patients presenting to the emergency department with unclassified ankle sprains. It failed to find a significant difference in pain or function within the first month comparing a PRP injection with a placebo injection.[24] Pain regimens and rehabilitation were not controlled. Further investigation is needed to determine if there is a role for PRP in acute lateral ankle or high ankle sprains.

Plantar fasciitis
Two meta-analyses comparing PRP with local steroid injections in recalcitrant plantar fasciitis were published in 2017. Yang and colleagues[25] reviewed 430 patients in 9 randomized control trials. There was no significant difference in the visual analog score improvements between the PRP group and steroid group in the short term (2–4 weeks) or intermediate term (4–8 weeks); however, the PRP group showed greater improvement compared with the steroid group in the long term (beyond 24 weeks). There were no differences in the Foot and Ankle Disability Index, American Orthopedic Foot and Ankle Society (AOFAS) scale, and Roles and Maudsley score between the PRP and steroid group. Singh and colleagues[26] reported on 517 patients in 10 randomized control trials, and found superior improvements in visual analog scores and AOFAS scores for PRP compared with steroid injections at the 3-month follow-up. There was no difference between the groups at 1-, 6-, or 12-month follow-ups.

The current evidence suggests that PRP may have equivocal outcomes to corticosteroid injections in the short term. Some authors have recommended use of PRP over steroids owing to reported long-term effectiveness.[25,27,28] In addition, PRP may avoid the known risks associated with corticosteroid injection, such as plantar fascia rupture;[29] however, more information is needed on relative rates of adverse events.[26] Cost-effectiveness of PRP must also be considered because average per-patient charges have been reported to be upward of $1500 per injection.[1]

Amniotic-Derived Products
Another recent area of interest is the use of amniotic tissue to enhance soft tissue healing. The amniotic membrane can be harvested from a placenta delivered by a cesarean section, thereby gaining pluripotent cell characteristics and avoiding the ethical debate surrounding use of human embryonic stem cells. Amniotic tissue has low immunogenicity and has been shown to inhibit inflammation, fibrosis, scarring, and microbial growth.[30]

Because of these beneficial properties, there has been recent interest in the use of amniotic membrane-human mesenchymal stromal cells in foot and ankle pathology. Although use of amniotic membrane-human mesenchymal stromal cells has been reported to be safe,[31,32] literature on its efficacy is sparse. In 2013, a level I prospective, randomized feasibility study was published comparing micronized dehydrated amniotic/chorionic membrane allograft and saline injections for plantar fasciitis. Patients receiving the allograft injection had significantly improved AOFAS scores at 1 and 8 weeks (P<.001).[33] Another level I prospective, randomized pilot trial reported that cryopreserved human amniotic membrane injections may be comparable with corticosteroid injections.[32] Both studies highlighted the need for future prospective trials with larger patient populations. Other studies currently available lack control groups and have risk for bias.[34–36] The current literature should be interpreted with caution because all of the studies discussed above have industry funding and/or author affiliation. At this point, no recommendation for use of amniotic-derived products in the foot and ankle can be made (**Fig. 3**).

ARTICULAR CARTILAGE

Microfracture is historically the standard first-line surgical treatment of many osteochondral lesions of the talus, particularly for those less than 1.5 cm^2.[37] However, extensive effort has been put forth in a quest to restore durable hyaline-like cartilage. Research is being conducted to elucidate the efficacy and durability of a multitude of treatment options including autologous chondrocyte and osteochondral implantation, matrix-induced autologous chondrocyte implantation, autologous matrix-induced chondrogenesis, fresh osteochondral allograft transplantation, matrix-associated stem cell transplantation, particulated juvenile cartilage allografts (PJCAs), bone marrow aspirate concentrate (BMAC), and PRP. A complex interplay between the host and lesion characteristics influences the likelihood of success with each treatment option.[38,39] A review of all the aforementioned treatments is beyond the scope of this paper. Following is a discussion of evidence behind adjunct orthobiologic options in the current literature.

Bone Marrow Aspirate Concentrate

Bone marrow-derived mesenchymal stem cells (MSCs) are capable of both chondrogenic and osteogenic differentiation *in vitro*.[40,41] Bone marrow aspirate may be harvested from the iliac crest, proximal tibia, distal tibia, or calcaneus; however, the iliac crest has been shown to have a higher concentration of osteoprogenitor cells compared with the distal tibia or calcaneus.[42] The retrieved aspirate is centrifuged to form BMAC, increasing the ratio of MSCs.[43] BMAC is also rich in growth factors and cytokines that help modulate differentiation, proliferation, and inflammatory response.[43,44] Attention has therefore been placed on using BMAC for osteochondral lesions, either with a biologic scaffold (matrix-associated stem cell transplantation), or as an adjunct to chondral and osteochondral grafts.[39,45,46]

The efficacy of BMAC for chondral defects is currently being explored in the orthopedic literature.[47] A 2017 systematic review of BMAC outcomes in talar osteochondral

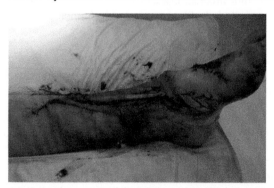

Fig. 3. Allografts minimize donor morbidity. Further research is needed to validate the use of various amniotic-derived grafts for use in complex traumatic wounds such as this pediatric patient with a degloving injury.

lesions reviewed 184 patients with a mean follow-up of 34 months.[45] The 4 studies available for inclusion in this review had significant heterogeneity, and used BMAC in varying capacities: as an adjunct to microfracture, augmenting autologous osteochondral transplant, or with arthroscopic debridement alone. Patient selection, lesion size, BMAC processing, and outcome measures varied greatly.[40,48–50] Overall, BMAC application in joints seems to be safe, and the reported complications in this review are consistent with known complications of the primary surgical intervention (donor site pain in patients who have undergone autologous osteochondral transplant, subchondral cysts, superficial peroneal nerve injuries, and a superficial infection at an arthroscopic portal site). Reporting efficacy is difficult, as 3 of the included studies were case series and 1 was a retrospective cohort. In these preliminary studies, positive results have been reported; however, the durability of repair is questioned. After BMAC administration with a biologic scaffold, Giannini and colleagues[50] observed a significant increase in AOFAS scores until 24 months postoperatively; however, they observed a relative decrease in AOFAS scores from 24- to 48 month postoperatively.

A recent prospective cohort study examining the use of arthroscopic microfracture alone (52 patients) versus microfracture with BMAC (49 patients) demonstrated a decreased need for revision arthroscopy when BMAC was used (29% revision rate for microfracture alone, 12% revision rate for microfracture and BMAC, $P = .0145$).[51] Most of the lesions in that study were small, between 0.7 and 1.5 cm². The reason for failure with microfracture alone was reported to be fissuring of the fibrocartilage with residual edema. Hannon and colleagues[49] also reported less fissuring and fibrillation on MRI in patients who received BMAC in addition to undergoing microfracture as compared with those who underwent microfracture alone; however, clinical outcomes were similar between the 2 groups.

Of note, hypertrophic growth of cartilage has been reported in up to 45% of patients receiving a second look arthroscopy or postoperative MRI.[40,50] This should be further investigated in future studies.

Platelet-Rich Plasma

The multitude of growth factors and cytokines in PRP stimulate MSCs, chondrocytes, and cellular proliferation, and certain preparations counter inflammation *in vivo*.[4,52,53] LP-PRP has shown efficacy in improving osteoarthritic symptoms in the literature on the orthopedic knee.[4] Limited research is available trialing its use in osteochondral lesions and osteoarthritis of the ankle. However, preliminary results have suggested positive results with intra-articular injections alone and in conjunction with microfracture.[54–57] Larger controlled studies are needed to further evaluate these preliminary clinical findings.

Hyaluronic Acid

Hyaluronic acid (HA) injections have been studied extensively in knee osteoarthritis; however, there is still debate regarding preparation and frequency of injections for optimal results.[58] HA use in joints is reported to be safe, although up to 15% of patients may have mild adverse effects (most commonly transient postinjection pain, especially with high-molecular-weight HA).[59] There have been reported positive results using HA for ankle osteoarthritis and osteochondral lesions;[59–63] however, intra-articular placebo effect may account for 87% of observed improvement.[59] Randomized controlled trials of HA use in ankle arthritis have not shown a significant advantage over saline injections or physical therapy, with the exception of Cohen and colleagues[64] finding a significant advantage to HA over saline at the 3-month mark.[64–67] As discussed by Abate and colleagues,[68] HA in relation to (1) osteoarthritic grade, (2) patient population, (3) dose regimen, and (4) outcome measures needs to be further investigated before abandoning the idea of HA in ankle osteoarthritis.

Particulated Juvenile Cartilage Allografts

PJCAs have been explored as a single-stage procedure for osteochondral lesions in the ankle.[69] Emphasis has been placed on obtaining grafts from juvenile donors because the chondrogenic potential is significantly higher in cells from donors younger than 13 years old.[70] PJCAs are reported to be best suited for lesions between 1 and 1.5 cm^2; however, the depth of the lesion and concomitant bone grafting confound results.[71,72] Retrospective studies have reported positive results.[72–75] However, a 2017 systematic review of PJCAs for osteochondral lesions of the talus showed an 84% success rate, which is comparable with reported rates for debridement and microfracture alone.[37,73] In addition, Karnovsky and colleagues[76] found no functional advantages comparing PJCAs with microfracture, although their supplemental use of BMAC in some microfracture patients complicates the interpretation of results. Postoperative MRI findings in patients who have undergone PJCA have shown fibrocartilage-like features, persistent chondral defects, hypertrophy, and subchondral edema, even up to 2 years postoperatively.[73,75,76] As with many other emerging orthobiologic techniques, the current literature has significant heterogeneity with regard to patient population, lesion characteristics, and technique. Overall, the level and quality of evidence is limited.[77] Evidence from prospective, randomized controlled trials is needed before PJCAs can be recommended for routine use.

Extracellular Matrix Cartilage Allografts

Extracellular matrix cartilage allografts contain micronized cartilage matrix and growth factors to act as a scaffold and promote the differentiation of stem cells into hyaline cartilage.[46,77] Although the theory has potential, there is, as yet, insufficient *in vitro* literature to support its use.[77,78]

BONE

The science of orthobiologics in bone healing is a complex and dynamic field. All products provide at least 1 of 3 major properties: osteoconduction, osteoinduction, or osteogenesis. Osteoconduction is the process by which a scaffold supports ingrowth of host cells required for osteogenesis; osteoinduction is the stimulation of host stem cells to differentiate into osteoprogenitor cells; and osteogenesis is the ability of the graft cells themselves to form new bone.[79,80] Autografting has long been held as the gold standard for bone grafting because it includes all 3 of these properties and has no risk of disease transmission.[81] Grafts can be harvested from multiple anatomic sites with overall low morbidity.[82–85] However, owing to concerns regarding donor site complications, longer operating time, and feasibility when a large volume is needed, a multitude of other options have been explored.[80,86,87] Allografting has been shown to provide sufficient osteoconductive properties and structural support; for example, in deformity correction, arthrodesis, or large traumatic bone defects.[88,89] Synthetic substitutes such as calcium phosphate, coralline hydroxyapatite, and bioactive glass are also used for osteoconductive scaffolds.[80] Demineralized bone matrix is an option for filling bone voids or augmenting fusion sites, providing osteoconductive and, to some degree, osteoinductive properties (**Fig. 4**).[80]

In poor host environments an emphasis is placed on optimizing osteoinductive properties. Osteoinductive cells can be concentrated from the host, for example, with BMAC and PRP, or developed into recombinant agents. Platelet-derived growth

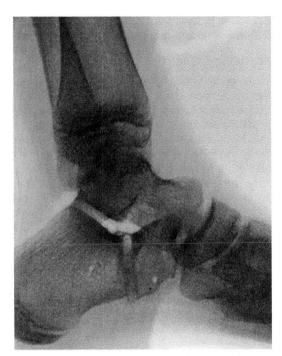

Fig. 4. Lengthening calcaneal osteotomy with allograft to provide structural support.

factor and bone morphogenic proteins (BMPs) both have recombinant forms that have been explored in the orthopedic literature.[79] Recently, bone grafts have been developed with the ability to preserve MSCs and growth factors through processing,[90,91] thereby obtaining osteoconductive, osteoinductive, and osteogenic properties from an allograft (**Fig. 5**).

There are many combinations possible for synergistic use of orthobiologic agents. In addition, there are a multitude of potential surgical uses and host environments. As with the broader literature on orthobiologics, this heterogeneity complicates interpretation of results and determination of indications. An overview of the clinical evidence, or in some cases a paucity of evidence, for these products follows.

Bone Marrow Aspirate Concentrate

Similar to its use in joints, BMAC has been used in fractures and nonunions, in part because of its ability to deliver growth factors and stem cells with osteogenic potential

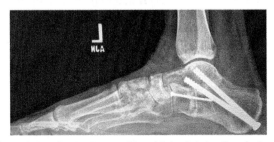

Fig. 5. Lengthening calcaneal osteotomy with subtalar joint arthrodesis and gastrocnemius recession for management of talocalcaneal coalition with hindfoot valgus.

directly to the fracture site.[87,92] It is often used in conjunction with an osteoconductive scaffold to keep the BMAC liquid at the desired location.[79] In foot and ankle literature, BMAC has been used in small cohorts of athletes with Jones fractures of the fifth metatarsal.[93–96] Although the investigators reported functional results, no conclusions regarding accelerated return to play or risk of refracture with BMAC versus fixation alone can be made at this time. However, BMAC may be indicated in certain subsets of patients who are at high risk. Hernigou and colleagues[97,98] found a higher rate of union and lower complication rates with use of BMAC compared with iliac crest autografts in diabetic patients undergoing surgery for a nonunion ankle fracture. The efficacy of BMAC in fracture healing may be influenced by the site of harvest, because bone healing rates are associated with concentration of MSCs.[97]

Platelet-Rich Plasma

The osteoinductive properties of PRP may have positive effects on bone healing.[79] It has been suggested that percutaneous injection of PRP or adjunct use during revision surgery increases healing rates of long bone nonunions.[99–101] Its use has also been explored as an adjunct to allografting in comminuted calcaneal fractures, in syndesmotic fusions, and in high-risk patients undergoing foot and ankle surgery.[102–105] There is potential for certain applications, especially in hosts with poor local healing sites; however, the use of PRP for osseous union is not yet well defined.

Bone Morphogenic Proteins

BMPs are growth factors that attract MSCs and initiate signaling pathways to induce osteogenesis and angiogenesis.[79,106] Two recombinant forms (rhBMP-2 and rhBMP-7) are available for use; however, they are not approved by the US Food and Drug Administration (FDA) for foot and ankle applications.[79] Concerns were raised in the literature on the spine regarding adverse reactions, including heterotopic ossification and possible carcinogenesis.[107,108] However, rhBMPs have been used off-label for use in ankle and rearfoot fusions.[109–113] The use of BMPs and their safety profile specific to foot and ankle surgery remains undefined. The FDA does warn against off-label use of BMPs in pediatric patients.[114]

Platelet-Derived Growth Factor

Platelet-derived growth factor (PDGF), a distinctly separate entity from PRP and platelet-rich growth factors (PRGFs), is released by platelets and plays an important role in angiogenesis and osteogenesis. The recombinant form rhPDGF-BB is an osteoinductive FDA-approved agent for foot and ankle arthrodesis.[87,115] rhPDGF-BB is often used with an osteoconductive agent, such as beta-tricalcium phosphate (B-TCP).[87,115] A large, prospective randomized controlled study by DiGiovanni and colleagues[116] found that rhPDGF-BB delivered through a scaffold of B-TCP was not inferior to use of an iliac crest autograft. They reported a satisfactory safety profile, with no statistically significant increase in adverse events for the rhPDGF-BB group compared with the autograft group, and predictably with an absence of donor site complications. There was no statistical difference in fusion rates between the rhPDGF-BB/B-TCP group and the autograft group (86.2% vs 87.6%, noninferiority $P = .008$).[116] Whereas there were early concerns regarding development of cancer with use of topical rhPDGF-BB, multiple clinical trials have found no association between the one-time surgical application of rhPDGF-BB and cancer incidence.[117] In 2018 the FDA approved use of rhPDGF-BB with an injectable mixture of B-TCP and bovine collagen matrix for use in hindfoot and ankle fusions.[118] The above studies were well designed and of high quality; however, it should be noted that they are all manufacturer funded.[116–118] Future studies should investigate the risk-benefit profile for rhDGF-BB with attention to cost and continued monitoring of adverse events.

Mesenchymal Stem Cell Allografts

Mesenchymal stem cell allografts (MSCAs) are relatively newer products and are differentiated by the fact that they contain viable osteogenic cells that are preserved through processing, thereby achieving osteoconductive, osteoinductive, and osteogenic properties. They can also be combined with demineralized cortical bone and B-TCP/collagen.[90,91] Retrospective studies have suggested efficacy in foot and ankle arthrodesis with 90% to 100% fusion rates in populations including high-risk patients.[119–123] A prospective study of MSCAs in foot and ankle fusion showed no major adverse events in a population of 92 patients 6 months postoperatively.[90] There were no significant differences in fusion rates with patients stratified by age or comorbidities, and the investigators hypothesized that the graft may mitigate the nonunion risk in higher-risk populations. This study was funded by the manufacturer and the investigators acknowledge that a randomized control trial is necessary to further investigate their outcomes.[90] MSCAs have also been described with the addition of BMAC.[124] Prospective trials focusing on the risk-benefit profile including fusion rates, adverse reactions, and cost profile of autograft versus MSCA are warranted.

Use in pediatrics

Structural bone grafting is used in reconstructive pediatric foot surgery.[125–127] Use of allografts may save operating room time and cost, and prevents donor site morbidity.[126,128] Risk of transmission of viral pathogens from allograft use is extremely low.[80,129]

Vining and colleagues[126] compared 182 structural allografts to 63 autografts in 161 pediatric patients undergoing reconstructive foot surgery. They found no statistical difference in time to graft union for the allograft compared with the autograft group (7.2 vs 7.4 weeks, $P = .45$). There was no graft rejection, collapse, deep infections, or transmission of viral pathogens. Nowicki and colleagues[127] examined complications and graft incorporation in 31 pediatric patients undergoing foot reconstruction with use of allografts, most of whom had an underlying neuromuscular disease. Twenty-eight grafts showed complete incorporation by 9 months, and the remaining 3 were lost to follow-up. There were 2 reported complications: 1 superficial wound dehiscence and 1 graft dislodgement. The investigators concluded that allografts were safe to use in pediatric foot surgery in patients with neuromuscular disease. Of note is the drastic difference in reported time to graft incorporation between the 2 studies discussed above (7 weeks vs 9 months). This is likely due to differences in radiographic assessment of allograft incorporation between investigators, and the inherent difficulty in radiographically assessing graft-host interfaces.[126] However, a slower incorporation owing to the underlying comorbidities in the Nowicki study cannot be excluded. The use of xenografts in pediatric flatfoot reconstruction is not recommended.[130] Currently the use of porous titanium wedges is being explored, which may provide another option besides autografts or allografts.[131] Further research is needed to assess the radiographic correction and long-term results with use of titanium wedges in adults and children (**Fig. 6**).

The use of osteoinductive agents in pediatric foot and ankle surgery is less clear. Due to a lower rate of host compromise from comorbidities, such as smoking or uncontrolled diabetes mellitus, their use is rarely indicated. The FDA warns against use of bone graft substitutes containing recombinant proteins or synthetic peptides in pediatric patients.[114] However, rhBMP has been used off-label in pediatric spine

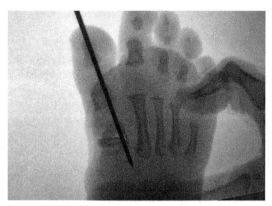

Fig. 6. Resection of longitudinal epiphyseal bracket in toddler. Allograft used for structural support.

surgery and congenital tibial pseudarthrosis.[51] The use of PRP in pediatric patients is currently being explored, and BMAC has been suggested for use in juvenile osteochondritis dissecans of the talus.[1,132]

Although limited, the current literature supports the use of structural allografts for pediatric foot surgery. Further investigation is needed to assess safety and efficacy of other osteobiologics, specifically with osteoinductive agents.

SUMMARY

The use of orthobiologics in foot and ankle pathology is an exciting field with significant potential. However, many available products lack peer-reviewed evidence, and, for those that do, the literature has high variation in techniques, study populations, and outcome measures. This leads to conflicting results that may obscure the true indications for respective products. Recent systematic reviews of PRP and BMAC in clinical orthopedic literature found that only 16% of articles on PRP and 14% of articles on BMAC quantitatively reported the composition of the final product.[45] No studies on BMAC and only 10% of studies on PRP provided a reproducible preparation technique in their methods.[45] Various classification systems have been suggested to standardize future PRP trials.[5,133–135] This act of standardizing the reporting of technique and results should be applied to all orthobiologic products, allowing for a clearer interpretation of their true efficacy. A focus should be maintained on completing large, high-quality prospective trials to elucidate the true indications for all emerging orthobiologic products in the foot and ankle.

It is important to recognize the concerns and unknown long-term reactions with utilization of osteogenic or osteoinductive products in the use of pediatrics. Children developing and undergoing osseous maturation may respond very differently to these products. At present, structural allografts are FDA approved in pediatric surgery, but ongoing research is needed to support further products.

REFERENCES

1. Zhang JY, Fabricant PD, Ishmael CR, et al. Utilization of platelet-rich plasma for musculoskeletal injuries. Orthop J Sports Med 2016;4(12):1–7.
2. Rodeo SA. Biologic approaches in sports medicine. Am J Sports Med 2016; 44(7):1657–9.

3. Hadley CJ, Shi WJ, Murphy H, et al. The clinical evidence behind biologic therapies promoted at annual orthopaedic meetings: a systematic review. Arthroscopy 2019;35(1):251–9.

4. Le AD, Enweze L, Debaun MR, et al. Platelet-rich plasma. Clin Sports Med 2019; 38(1):17–44.

5. Mishra A, Harmon K, Woodall J, et al. Sports medicine applications of platelet rich plasma. Curr Pharm Biotechnol 2012;13(7):1185–95.

6. Anitua E, Andia I, Ardanza B, et al. Autologous platelets as a source of proteins for healing and tissue regeneration. Thromb Haemost 2004;91(01):4–15.

7. Di Matteo D, Filardo G, Kon E, et al. Platelet-rich plasma: evidence for the treatment of patellar and Achilles tendinopathy—a systematic review. Musculoskelet Surg 2014;99(1):1–9.

8. De Vos RJ, Weir A, Tol JL, et al. No effects of PRP on ultrasonographic tendon structure and neovascularisation in chronic midportion Achilles tendinopathy. Br J Sports Med 2010;45(5):387–92.

9. De Jonge S, Vos RJD, Weir A, et al. One-year follow-up of platelet-rich plasma treatment in chronic Achilles tendinopathy. Am J Sports Med 2011;39(8):1623–30.

10. Krogh TP, Ellingsen T, Christensen R, et al. Ultrasound-guided injection therapy of Achilles tendinopathy with platelet-rich plasma or saline. Am J Sports Med 2016;44(8):1990–7.

11. Boesen AP, Hansen R, Boesen MI, et al. Effect of high-volume injection, platelet-rich plasma, and sham treatment in chronic midportion Achilles tendinopathy: a randomized double-blinded prospective study. Am J Sports Med 2017;45(9):2034–43.

12. Zhang YJ, Xu SZ, Gu PC, et al. Is platelet-rich plasma injection effective for chronic Achilles tendinopathy? A meta-analysis. Clin Orthop Relat Res 2018;476:1633–41.

13. Yeo A, Kendall N, Jayaraman S. Ultrasound-guided dry needling with percutaneous paratenon decompression for chronic Achilles tendinopathy. Knee Surg Sports Traumatol Arthrosc 2014;24(7):2112–8.

14. Chan O, O'Dowd D, Padhiar N, et al. High volume image guided injections in chronic Achilles tendinopathy. Disabil Rehabil 2008;30(20–22):1697–708.

15. Sadoghi P, Rosso C, Valderrabano V, et al. The role of platelets in the treatment of Achilles tendon injuries. J Orthop Res 2012;31(1):111–8.

16. Alsousou J, Thompson M, Harrison P, et al. Effect of platelet-rich plasma on healing tissues in acute ruptured Achilles tendon: a human immunohistochemistry study. Lancet 2015;385:S19.

17. De Carli A, Lanzetti RM, Ciompi A, et al. Can platelet-rich plasma have a role in Achilles tendon surgical repair? Knee Surg Sports Traumatol Arthrosc 2015; 24(7):2231–7.

18. Kaniki N, Willits K, Mohtadi NG, et al. A retrospective comparative study with historical control to determine the effectiveness of platelet-rich plasma as part of nonoperative treatment of acute Achilles tendon rupture. Arthroscopy 2014; 30(9):1139–45.

19. Schepull T, Kvist J, Norrman H, et al. Autologous platelets have no effect on the healing of human Achilles tendon ruptures. Am J Sports Med 2011;39(1):38–47.

20. Zou J, Mo X, Shi Z, et al. A prospective study of platelet-rich plasma as biological augmentation for acute Achilles tendon rupture repair. Biomed Res Int 2016; 2016:1–8.

21. Sánchez M, Anitua E, Azofra J, et al. Comparison of surgically repaired Achilles tendon tears using platelet-rich fibrin matrices. Am J Sports Med 2007;35(2):245–51.

22. Laver L, Carmont MR, Mcconkey MO, et al. Plasma rich in growth factors (PRGF) as a treatment for high ankle sprain in elite athletes: a randomized control trial. Knee Surg Sports Traumatol Arthrosc 2014;23(11):3383–92.

23. Samra DJ, Sman AD, Rae K, et al. Effectiveness of a single platelet-rich plasma injection to promote recovery in rugby players with ankle syndesmosis injury. BMJ Open Sport Exerc Med 2015;1(1):e000033.

24. Rowden A, Dominici P, Dorazio J, et al. Double-blind, randomized, placebo-controlled study evaluating the use of platelet-rich plasma therapy (PRP) for acute ankle sprains in the emergency department. J Emerg Med 2015;49(4): 546–51.

25. Yang W, Han Y, Cao X, et al. Platelet-rich plasma as a treatment for plantar fasciitis. A meta-analysis of randomized controlled trials. Medicine 2017; 96(44):1–8.

26. Singh P, Madanipour S, Bhamra JS, et al. A systematic review and meta-analysis of platelet-rich plasma versus corticosteroid injections for plantar fasciopathy. Int Orthop 2017;41(6):1169–81.

27. Monto RR. Platelet-rich plasma efficacy versus corticosteroid injection treatment for chronic severe plantar fasciitis. Foot Ankle Int 2014;35(4):313–8.

28. Jain K, Murphy PN, Clough TM. Platelet rich plasma versus corticosteroid injection for plantar fasciitis: a comparative study. Foot 2015;25(4):235–7.

29. Acevedo JI, Beskin JL. Complications of plantar fascia rupture associated with corticosteroid injection. Foot Ankle Int 1998;19(2):91–7.

30. Niknejad H, Peirovi H, Jorjani M, et al. Properties of the amniotic membrane for potential use in tissue engineering. Eur Cell Mater 2008;7:88–99.

31. DeMill SL, Granata JD, McAlister JE, et al. Safety analysis of cryopreserved amniotic membrane/umbilical cord tissue in foot and ankle surgery: a consecutive case series of 124 patients. Surg Technol Int 2014;25:257–61.

32. Hanselman AE, Tidwell JE, Santrock RD. Cryopreserved human amniotic membrane injection for plantar fasciitis. Foot Ankle Int 2015;36(2):151–8.

33. Zelen CM, Poka A, Andrews J. Prospective, randomized, blinded, comparative study of injectable micronized dehydrated amniotic/chorionic membrane allograft for plantar fasciitis—a feasibility study. Foot Ankle Int 2013;34(10):1332–9.

34. Werber B. Amniotic tissues for the treatment of chronic plantar fasciosis and Achilles tendinosis. J Sports Med 2015;2015:1–6.

35. Warner M, Lasyone L. An open-label, single-center, retrospective study of cryopreserved amniotic membrane and umbilical cord tissue as an adjunct for foot and ankle surgery. Surg Technol Int 2014;25:251–5.

36. Lullove E. A flowable placental tissue matrix allograft in lower extremity injuries: a pilot study. Cureus 2015;7(6):e275.

37. Zengerink M, Struijs PAA, Tol JL, et al. Treatment of osteochondral lesions of the talus: a systematic review. Knee Surg Sports Traumatol Arthrosc 2009;18(2): 238–46.

38. Mcgoldrick N, Murphy E, Kearns S. Osteochondral lesions of the ankle: the current evidence supporting scaffold-based techniques and biological adjuncts. Foot Ankle Surg 2018;24(2):86–91.

39. Kraeutler MJ, Chahla J, Dean CS, et al. Current concepts review update. Foot Ankle Int 2017;38(3):331–42.

40. Giannini S, Buda R, Vannini F, et al. One-step bone marrow-derived cell transplantation in talar osteochondral lesions. Clin Orthop Relat Res 2009;467(12): 3307–20.

41. Pittenger MF. Multilineage potential of adult human mesenchymal stem cells. Science 1999;284(5411):143–7.
42. Hyer CF, Berlet GC, Bussewitz BW, et al. Quantitative assessment of the yield of osteoblastic connective tissue progenitors in bone marrow aspirate from the iliac crest, tibia, and calcaneus. J Bone Joint Surg Am 2013;95(14):1312–6.
43. Holton J, Imam M, Ward J, et al. The basic science of bone marrow aspirate concentrate in chondral injuries. Orthop Rev 2016;8(3).
44. Cassano JM, Kennedy JG, Ross KA, et al. Bone marrow concentrate and platelet-rich plasma differ in cell distribution and interleukin 1 receptor antagonist protein concentration. Knee Surg Sports Traumatol Arthrosc 2016;26(1): 333–42.
45. Chahla J, Cinque ME, Schon JM, et al. Bone marrow aspirate concentrate for the treatment of osteochondral lesions of the talus: a systematic review of outcomes. J Exp Orthop 2016;3(33):33.
46. Shieh AK, Singh SG, Nathe C, et al. Effects of micronized cartilage matrix on cartilage repair in osteochondral lesions of the talus. Cartilage 2018;2(3):1–7.
47. Southworth TM, Naveen NB, Nwachukwu BU, et al. Orthobiologics for focal articular cartilage defects. Clin Sports Med 2019;38(1):109–22.
48. Kennedy JG, Murawski CD. The treatment of osteochondral lesions of the talus with autologous osteochondral transplantation and bone marrow aspirate concentrate. Cartilage 2011;2(4):327–36.
49. Hannon CP, Ross KA, Murawski CD, et al. Arthroscopic bone marrow stimulation and concentrated bone marrow aspirate for osteochondral lesions of the talus: a case-control study of functional and magnetic resonance observation of cartilage repair tissue outcomes. Arthroscopy 2016;32(2):339–47.
50. Giannini S, Buda R, Battaglia M, et al. One-step repair in talar osteochondral lesions. Am J Sports Med 2013;41(3):511–8.
51. Murphy E, McGoldrick N, Curtin M, et al. A prospective evaluation of bone marrow aspirate concentrate and microfracture in the treatment of osteochondral lesions of the talus. Foot Ankle Surg 2018. https://doi.org/10.1016/j.fas. 2018.02.011.
52. Smyth NA. Establishing proof of concept: platelet-rich plasma and bone marrow aspirate concentrate may improve cartilage repair following surgical treatment for osteochondral lesions of the talus. World J Orthop 2012;3(7):101.
53. Van Buul GM, Koevoet WL, Kops N, et al. Platelet-rich plasma releasate inhibits inflammatory processes in osteoarthritic chondrocytes. Am J Sports Med 2011; 39(11):2362–70.
54. Repetto I, Biti B, Cerruti P, et al. Conservative treatment of ankle osteoarthritis: can platelet-rich plasma effectively postpone surgery? J Foot Ankle Surg 2017;56(2):362–5.
55. Mei-Dan O, Carmont MR, Laver L, et al. Platelet-rich plasma or hyaluronate in the management of osteochondral lesions of the talus. Am J Sports Med 2012;40(3):534–41.
56. Görmeli G, Karakaplan M, Görmeli CA, et al. Clinical effects of platelet-rich plasma and hyaluronic acid as an additional therapy for talar osteochondral lesions treated with microfracture surgery. Foot Ankle Int 2015;36(8):891–900.
57. Guney A, Akar M, Karaman I, et al. Clinical outcomes of platelet rich plasma (PRP) as an adjunct to microfracture surgery in osteochondral lesions of the talus. Knee Surg Sports Traumatol Arthrosc 2013;23(8):2384–9.
58. Yaftali N, Weber K. Corticosteroids and hyaluronic acid injections. Clin Sports Med 2019;38:1–15.

59. Chang KV, Hsiao MY, Chen WS, et al. Effectiveness of intra-articular hyaluronic acid for ankle osteoarthritis treatment: a systematic review and meta-analysis. Arch Phys Med Rehabil 2013;94:951–60.

60. Carpenter B, Motley T. The role of viscosupplementation in the ankle using Hylan G-F 20. J Foot Ankle Surg 2008;47(5):377–84.

61. Sun S-F, Chou Y-J, Hsu C-W, et al. Efficacy of intra-articular hyaluronic acid in patients with osteoarthritis of the ankle: a prospective study. Osteoarthritis Cartilage 2006;14(9):867–74.

62. Mei-Dan O, Maoz G, Swartzon M, et al. Treatment of osteochondritis dissecans of the ankle with hyaluronic acid injections: a prospective study. Foot Ankle Int 2008;29(12):1171–8.

63. Han SH, Park DY, Kim TH. Prognostic factors after intra-articular hyaluronic acid injection in ankle osteoarthritis. Yonsei Med J 2014;55(4):1080.

64. Cohen MM, Altman RD, Hollstrom R, et al. Safety and efficacy of intra-articular sodium Hyaluronate (Hyalgan®) in a randomized, double-blind study for osteoarthritis of the ankle. Foot Ankle Int 2008;29(7):657–63.

65. DeGroot H, Uzunishvili S, Weir R, et al. Intra-articular injection of hyaluronic acid is not superior to saline solution injection for ankle arthritis. J Bone Joint Surg Am 2012;94:2–8.

66. Salk RS, Chang TJ, D'costa WF, et al. Sodium hyaluronate in the treatment of osteoarthritis of the ankle. J Bone Joint Surgery Am 2006;88(2):295–302.

67. Karatosun V, Unver B, Ozden A, et al. Intra-articular hyaluronic acid compared to exercise therapy in osteoarthritis of the ankle. Clin Exp Rheumatol 2008;26:288–94.

68. Abate M, Schiavone C, Salini V. Hyaluronic acid in ankle osteoarthritis: why evidence of efficacy is still lacking? Clin Exp Rheumatol 2012;30:277–81.

69. Ng A, Bernhard K. The use of particulated juvenile allograft cartilage in foot and ankle surgery. Clin Podiatr Med Surg 2018;35(1):11–8.

70. Adkisson HD, Martin JA, Amendola RL, et al. The potential of human allogeneic juvenile chondrocytes for restoration of articular cartilage. Am J Sports Med 2010;38(7):1324–33.

71. Dekker T, Hamid K, Easley M, et al. Efficacy of particulated juvenile cartilage allograft transplantation for osteochondral lesions of the talus. Foot Ankle Int 2017;39(3):278–83.

72. Coetzee JC, Giza E, Schon L, et al. Treatment of osteochondral lesions of the talus with particulated juvenile cartilage. Foot Ankle Int 2013;34(9):1205–11.

73. Saltzman BM, Lin J, Lee S. Particulated juvenile articular cartilage allograft transplantation for osteochondral talar lesions. Cartilage 2017;8(1):61–72.

74. Lanham NS, Carroll JJ, Cooper MT, et al. A comparison of outcomes of particulated juvenile articular cartilage and bone marrow aspirate concentrate for articular cartilage lesions of the talus. Foot Ankle Spec 2016;10(4):315–21.

75. Desandis BA, Haleem AM, Sofka CM, et al. Arthroscopic treatment of osteochondral lesions of the talus using juvenile articular cartilage allograft and autologous bone marrow aspirate concentration. J Foot Ankle Surg 2018;57(2):273–80.

76. Karnovsky SC, DeSandis B, Haleem A, et al. Comparison of juvenile allogenous articular cartilage and bone marrow aspirate concentrate versus microfracture with and without bone marrow aspirate concentrate in arthroscopic treatment of talar osteochondral lesions. Foot Ankle Int 2018;39(4):393–405.

77. Seow D, Yasui Y, Hurley ET, et al. Extracellular matrix cartilage allograft and particulate cartilage allograft for osteochondral lesions of the knee and ankle joints: a systematic review. Am J Sports Med 2017;46(7):1758–66.

78. Dekker R, Patel M. Outcomes of surgical treatment of talar osteochondral lesions using bone marrow aspirate and microgenized allograft cartilage extracellular matrix. Foot Ankle Int 2018;3(3). https://doi.org/10.1177/2473011418S00210.

79. Calcei JG, Rodeo SA. Orthobiologics for bone healing. Clin Sports Med 2019;38(1):79–95.

80. Finkemeier CG. Bone-grafting and bone-graft substitutes. J Bone Joint Surg Am 2002;84(3):454–64.

81. Miller CP, Chiodo CP. Autologous bone graft in foot and ankle surgery. Foot Ankle Clin 2016;21(4):825–37.

82. Danziger MB, Abdo RV, Decker JE. Distal tibia bone graft for arthrodesis of the foot and ankle. Foot Ankle Int 1995;16(4):187–90.

83. Deorio JK, Farber DC. Morbidity associated with anterior iliac crest bone grafting in foot and ankle surgery. Foot Ankle Int 2005;26(2):147–51.

84. Geideman W, Early JS, Brodsky J. Clinical results of harvesting autogenous cancellous graft from the ipsilateral proximal tibia for use in foot and ankle surgery. Foot Ankle Int 2004;25(7):451–5.

85. Singleton TJ, Schuberth JM. Bone graft from the distal medial tibia in foot and ankle surgery. Foot Ankle Spec 2012;5(3):168–74.

86. O'Malley MJ, Sayres SC, Saleem O, et al. Morbidity and complications following percutaneous calcaneal autograft bone harvest. Foot Ankle Int 2013;35(1):30–7.

87. Yeoh JC, Taylor BA. Osseous healing in foot and ankle surgery with autograft, allograft, and other orthobiologics. Orthop Clin North Am 2017;48(3):359–69.

88. Myerson MS, Neufeld SK, Uribe J. Fresh-frozen structural allografts in the foot and ankle. J Bone Joint Surg Am 2005;87(1):113–20.

89. Vosseller JT, Ellis SJ, O'Malley MJ, et al. Autograft and allograft unite similarly in lateral column lengthening for adult acquired flatfoot deformity. HSS J 2013;9(1):6–11.

90. Jones CP, Loveland J, Atkinson BL, et al. Prospective, multicenter evaluation of allogeneic bone matrix containing viable osteogenic cells in foot and/or ankle arthrodesis. Foot Ankle Int 2015;36(10):1129–37.

91. Rush SM. Trinity evolution. Foot Ankle Spec 2010;3(3):140–3.

92. Harford JS, Dekker TJ, Adams SB. Bone marrow aspirate concentrate for bone healing in foot and ankle surgery. Foot Ankle Clin 2016;21(4):839–45.

93. Murawski CD, Kennedy JG. Percutaneous internal fixation of proximal fifth metatarsal jones fractures (zones II and III) with Charlotte Carolina screw and bone marrow aspirate concentrate. Am J Sports Med 2011;39(6):1295–301.

94. Hunt KJ, Anderson RB. Treatment of jones fracture nonunions and refractures in the elite athlete. Am J Sports Med 2011;39(9):1948–54.

95. O'Malley M, Desandis B, Allen A, et al. Operative treatment of fifth metatarsal jones fractures (zones II and III) in the NBA. Foot Ankle Int 2016;37(5):488–500.

96. Carney D, Chambers MC, Kromka JJ, et al. Jones fracture in the elite athlete: patient reported outcomes following fixation with BMAC. Orthop J Sports Med 2018;6(7_suppl4).

97. Hernigou P, Guissou I, Homma Y, et al. Percutaneous injection of bone marrow mesenchymal stem cells for ankle non-unions decreases complications in patients with diabetes. Int Orthop 2015;39(8):1639–43.

98. Hernigou P, Poignard A, Beaujean F, et al. Percutaneous autologous bone-marrow grafting for nonunions. J Bone Joint Surg Am 2005;87(7):1430–7.

99. Malhotra R, Kumar V, Garg B, et al. Role of autologous platelet-rich plasma in treatment of long-bone nonunions: a prospective study. Musculoskelet Surg 2015;99(3):243–8.

100. Duramaz A, Ursavaş HT, Bilgili MG, et al. Platelet-rich plasma versus exchange intramedullary nailing in treatment of long bone oligotrophic nonunions. Eur J Orthop Surg Traumatol 2017;28(1):131–7.

101. Ghaffarpasand F, Shahrezaei M, Dehghankhalili M. Effects of platelet rich plasma on healing rate of long bone non-union fractures: a randomized double-blind placebo controlled clinical trial. Bull Emerg Trauma 2016;4(3):134–40.

102. Wei L-C, Lei G-H, Sheng P-Y, et al. Efficacy of platelet-rich plasma combined with allograft bone in the management of displaced intra-articular calcaneal fractures: a prospective cohort study. J Orthop Res 2012;30(10):1570–6.

103. Coetzee JC, Pomeroy GC, Watts JD, et al. The use of autologous concentrated growth factors to promote syndesmosis fusion in the agility total ankle replacement. a preliminary study. Foot Ankle Int 2005;26(10):840–6.

104. Bibbo C, Bono C, Lin S. Union rates using autologous platelet concentrate alone and with bone graft in high-risk foot and ankle surgery patients. J Surg Orthop Adv 2005;14(1):17–22.

105. Pinzur MS. Use of platelet-rich concentrate and bone marrow aspirate in high-risk patients with Charcot arthropathy of the foot. Foot Ankle Int 2009;30(02):124–7.

106. Zhao E, Carney D, Chambers M, et al. The role of biologic in foot and ankle trauma—a review of the literature. Curr Rev Musculoskelet Med 2018;11(3):495–502.

107. Fu R, Selph S, McDonagh M, et al. Effectiveness and harms of recombinant human bone morphogenetic protein-2 in spine fusion: a systematic review and meta-analysis. Ann Intern Med 2013;158(12):890–902.

108. Tannoury CA, An HS. Complications with the use of bone morphogenetic protein 2 (BMP-2) in spine surgery. Spine J 2014;14(3):552–9.

109. Fourman MS, Borst EW, Bogner E, et al. Recombinant human BMP-2 increases the incidence and rate of healing in complex ankle arthrodesis. Clin Orthop Relat Res 2013;472(2):732–9.

110. Kanakaris NK, Mallina R, Calori GM, et al. Use of bone morphogenetic proteins in arthrodesis: clinical results. Injury 2009;40(S3):S62–6.

111. Hernandez JLY, Abad J, Remy S, et al. Tibiotalocalcaneal arthrodesis using a straight intramedullary nail. Foot Ankle Int 2015;36(5):539–46.

112. Rearick T, Charlton TP, Thordarson D. Effectiveness and complications associated with recombinant human bone morphogenetic protein-2 augmentation of foot and ankle fusions and fracture nonunions. Foot Ankle Int 2014;35(8):783–8.

113. Schuberth JM, Didomenico LA, Mendicino RW. The utility and effectiveness of bone morphogenetic protein in foot and ankle surgery. J Foot Ankle Surg 2009;48(3):309–14.

114. Kestle JRW. Editorial: Food and Drug Administration safety communication on rhBMP-2 use. J Neurosurg Pediatr 2015;16(1):1–3.

115. Digiovanni CW, Petricek JM. The evolution of rhPDGF-BB in musculoskeletal repair and its role in foot and ankle fusion surgery. Foot Ankle Clin 2010;15(4):621–40.

116. DiGiovanni CW, Lin SS, Baumhauer JF, et al. Recombinant human platelet-derived growth factor-BB and beta-tricalcium phosphate (rhPDGF-BB/b-TCP): an alternative to autogenous bone graft. J Bone Joint Surg Am 2013;95:1184–92.

117. Solchaga LA, Hee CK, Roach S, et al. Safety of recombinant human platelet-derived growth factor-BB in augment bone graft. J Tissue Eng 2012;3(1):1–6.

118. Daniels TR, Younger ASE, Penner MJ, et al. Prospective randomized controlled trial of hindfoot and ankle fusions treated with rhPDGF-BB in combination with a β-TCP-Collagen Matrix. Foot Ankle Int 2015;36(7):739–48.

119. Rush SM, Hamilton GA, Ackerson LM. Mesenchymal stem cell allograft in revision foot and ankle surgery: a clinical and radiographic analysis. J Foot Ankle Surg 2009;48(2):163–9.

120. Scott RT, Hyer CF. Role of cellular allograft containing mesenchymal stem cells in high-risk foot and ankle reconstructions. J Foot Ankle Surg 2013;52(1):32–5.

121. Hollawell SM. Allograft cellular bone matrix as an alternative to autograft in hindfoot and ankle fusion procedures. J Foot Ankle Surg 2012;51(2):222–5.

122. Hollawell S, Kane B, Heisey C, et al. The role of allograft bone in foot and ankle arthrodesis and high-risk fracture management. Foot Ankle Spec 2018. https://doi.org/10.1177/1938640018815227.

123. Anderson J, Jeppesen N, Hansen M, et al. First metatarsophalangeal joint arthrodesis: comparison of mesenchymal stem cell allograft versus autogenous bone graft fusion rates. Surg Sci 2013;04(05):263–7.

124. Guyton GP, Miller SD. Stem cells in bone grafting: trinity allograft with stem cells and collagen/beta-tricalcium phosphate with concentrated bone marrow aspirate. Foot Ankle Clin 2010;15(4):611–9.

125. Mosca VS. Calcaneal lengthening for valgus deformity of the hindfoot. Results in children who had severe, symptomatic flatfoot and skewfoot. J Bone Joint Surg Am 1995;77(4):500–12.

126. Vining NC, Warme WJ, Mosca VS. Comparison of structural bone autografts and allografts in pediatric foot surgery. J Pediatr Orthop 2012;32(7):714–8.

127. Nowicki PD, Tylkowski CM, Iwinski HJ. Structural bone allograft in pediatric foot surgery. Am J Orthopedics 2010;39(5):238–40.

128. Skaggs D, Samuelson M, Hale J, et al. Complications of posterior iliac crest bone grafting in spine surgery in children. Spine 2000;25(18):2400–2.

129. Ng VY. Risk of disease transmission with bone allograft. Orthopedics 2012; 35(8):679–81.

130. Ledford CK, Nunley JA, Viens NA, et al. Bovine xenograft failures in pediatric foot reconstructive surgery. J Pediatr Orthop 2013;33(4):458–63.

131. Gross CE, Huh J, Gray J, et al. Radiographic outcomes following lateral column lengthening with a porous titanium wedge. Foot Ankle Int 2015;36(8):953–60.

132. Pagliazzi G, Baldassarri M, Perazzo L, et al. Tissue bioengineering in the treatment of osteochondritis dissecans of the talus in children with open physis. J Pediatr Orthop 2018;38(7):375–81.

133. Ehrenfest DMD, Rasmusson L, Albrektsson T. Classification of platelet concentrates: from pure platelet-rich plasma (P-PRP) to leucocyte- and platelet-rich fibrin (L-PRF). Trends Biotechnol 2009;27(3):158–67.

134. Delong JM, Russell RP, Mazzocca AD. Platelet-rich plasma: the PAW classification system. Arthroscopy 2012;28(7):998–1009.

135. Ehrenfest DMD, Andia I, Zumstein MA, et al. Classification of platelet concentrates (platelet-rich plasma-PRP, platelet-rich fibrin-PRF) for topical and infiltrative use in orthopedic and sports medicine: current consensus, clinical implications and perspectives. Muscles Ligaments Tendons J 2014;4(1):3–9.

Infection Protocols for Implants

Dena El-Sayed, MD[a], Aksone Nouvong, DPM[b],*

KEYWORDS

• Implants • Infection • Antibiotics • Prosthetic joint • Biofilm

KEY POINTS

• Prosthetic implant infections can form biofilms.
• Complications of prosthetic implants can lead to excessive antibiotic use, implant removal, reoperation, and potential amputation.
• Early recognition of implant infection is crucial.
• Antibiotic selection is imperative for optimization of treatment.
• Surgical treatment strategies can include debridement and retention, 1-stage or 2-stage exchange, permanent resection arthroplasty, arthrodesis, and amputation.

INTRODUCTION

In the United States, endoprosthetic procedures such as total knee arthroplasty (TKA), total hip arthroplasty (THA), and total ankle arthroplasty (TAA) are increasing and the number of revisional surgeries is concurrently increasing.[1] Infection can be a devastating complication of surgically inserted prosthetic implants. Trauma requiring prosthetic implants, including internal fixation devices (eg, plates, intramedullary nails), external fixation pins or screws, and prosthetic ankle, knee, and hip joint arthroplasty is common. Infections of these devices can lead to significant morbidity related to delayed healing and nonunion of the fracture, requiring multiple surgeries and revisions, and possibly even amputation.[2]

About 2-million implants were inserted in the United States in 2004,[3] and, despite appropriate perioperative antibiotics, approximately 5% of internal fixation devices became infected. The incidence of infection in revision surgery is high, with an estimated rate of 3.2% to 5.6% for both hips and knees. Infection accounts for as much as 12% of the indications for revision hip arthroplasty and 22% for revision

Disclosures: The authors have nothing to disclose.
[a] Internal Medicine Clinic, Infectious Diseases Clinic, Ventura County Medical Center, Ventura, CA, USA; [b] Department of Surgery, Division of Vascular Surgery, David Geffen School of Medicine at UCLA, 200 Medical Plaza, Suite 526, Los Angeles, CA 90095, USA
* Corresponding author.
E-mail address: anouvong@mednet.ucla.edu

knee arthroplasty.[4] A review of the current literature reports that the rate of infection for TAA ranges from 2.4% to 8.9%. These rates are greater than those for TKA and THA,[5] possibly because of the watershed area and frail soft tissue envelop surrounding the ankle, which predisposes the area to develop wound dehiscence and delayed wound healing.[6,7]

Recent studies have analyzed the occurrence and severity of prosthetic joint infections (PJI) associated with knee and hip arthroplasty. Kurtz and colleagues[8] found that the knee infection rate at 0.92% was significantly greater than that of hip arthroplasties, which was 0.88%. The rates of periprosthetic infections following revision of TKA are 3% to 5%. In Ruedi type III pilon fractures treated with early internal fixation, infection rates are up to 37%. Internal fixation of closed fractures have lower infection rates than open fractures, for which the infection rate can be as high as 22.7%.[9–12]

PJI can be categorized into early-onset, delayed-onset, and late-onset PJI, which are discussed further later.[1] Another described classification has been described as an infection identified only by positive intraoperative culture during routine revisional arthroplasty that was presumed to be aseptic loosening preoperatively.[7]

Several risk factors have been identified to increase the PJI risk, including longer surgical time and revisional surgery. Patients' comorbidities, including diabetes, low body mass index, obesity, inflammatory arthritis, peripheral vascular disease, hypothyroidism, and prior ankle surgery, were also strong confounding factors for infection risk. Infection secondary to multidrug resistance has increased over the years. Advanced age, history of antibiotic treatment, hospital admission, and living in a long-term-care facility are risk factors for infection of the urinary tract, respiratory system, and surgical wounds, including orthopedic devices.[5,13–15] These risk factors differ from those of TKA and THA, likely owing to a different population of patients undergoing TAA. TAA is often performed in patients who have sustained trauma rather than for osteoarthritis.[5]

There are significant numbers of studies examining the effectiveness of irrigation and debridement (I&D) with polyethylene exchange, and retention of the metal components in TAA, TKA, and THA. Some of the important predictors of failure include the duration of symptoms and the pathogenic bacterial species. Longer duration of symptoms, as well as the isolation of methicillin-resistant *Staphylococcus aureus* (MRSA), is associated with higher failure rates with I&D and polyethylene exchange. Although there are many discussions in the literature on TKA and THA, there is a paucity of studies on TAA.[1]

Radiographic findings are not consistently helpful because the postoperative scans are difficult to interpret, which is discussed further later.[11] Nuclear imaging techniques are often sensitive, but these imaging modalities have difficulty distinguishing between mechanical and infectious causes.[9,16] Cultures of the prosthetic implants have been reported to yield poor outcomes, but studies by Hyung-Jin Park and colleagues[17] showed a sensitivity of 92% when periprosthetic tissue was placed in blood culture bottles. In addition, molecular techniques have been used in the examination of PJI and have identified many pathogens, some with definite importance and others playing an uncertain role.

With both internal fixation devices and PJI, early infections are often caused by virulent organisms such as *S aureus*. Other organisms isolated, such as gram-negative organisms or anaerobes, may represent contamination or colonization and are not necessarily pathogenic. However, studies have shown that gram-negative organisms were isolated in high proportions of fracture-fixation devices,[18] and, in another study of 202 open fractures, at least 1 gram-negative organism was present in 55%.[19]

Therefore, if there is suspicion for prosthetic implant infection, it may be prudent to include gram-negative coverage in empiric antibiotic choices.

More than 65% of all human infections are biofilm related. Prosthetic joint and internal fixation device infections are often complicated by a biofilm, formed by bacteria secreting an extracellular polymeric substance, which results in an increase in false-negative cultures and poor penetration of antibiotics.[11] S aureus is the most common organism encountered in biofilms and strains of S aureus in biofilms are often drug resistant. Biofilm-forming strains are more frequently isolated from nonfluid tissues, particularly bone and soft tissues. Romanó and colleagues[20] point out that implant-related infections are complex, starting with bacterial adhesion in biofilm formation, followed by variable interactions between host implant microorganisms and their byproducts. Clinical presentations may differ, depending on the balance of these factors. The presence of bacterial biofilm may make detection of pathogens difficult when traditional microbiological techniques are used.[21] Sonication may be of value here, because it dislodges bacteria from biofilm and has been shown to increase the sensitivity of cultures in PJI.[22–27] A study by Esteban and colleagues[28–30] evaluated sonication of 4 intramedullary nails and 8 other osteosynthetic materials and showed a sensitivity of 94.7% from sonicate fluid culture, compared with a sensitivity of 84.2% from conventional cultures.

Strict collaboration between surgeons, infectious disease clinicians, microbiologist, pathologists, and radiologists is recommended in management of these infections. Early diagnosis and treatment are crucial to improve the postoperative outcome and salvaging of the prosthesis.

DIAGNOSIS
Definition

he Infectious Diseases Society of America (IDSA) published guidelines in 2012 delineating diagnostic criteria and management strategies for PJI. The guidelines are based primarily on data from hip and knee PJI but encompass diagnosis and management of prosthetic ankle and foot PJI. The criteria for definition of PJI from the IDSA guidelines are shown in **Box 1**, compared with the definition criteria developed by

---

Box 1
Infectious Diseases Society of America definition

1. Presence of a sinus tract that communicates with prosthesis is definitive evidence of PJI.

2. Acute inflammation seen on histopathologic examination of periprosthetic tissue at time of surgical debridement or prosthesis removal is highly suggestive evidence of PJI.

3. Presence of purulence surrounding a prosthesis without another known cause (eg, failed metal-on-metal arthroplasty) is definitive evidence of PJI.

4. Two or more intraoperative cultures/combination of preoperative aspiration and intraoperative culture that yield the same organisms may be considered definitive evidence of PJI.

5. Growth of virulent microorganism (ie, S aureus) in single specimen of tissue biopsy or synovial fluid may represent PJI. Growth of a common contaminant in multiple tissue cultures/single aspiration culture should be evaluated in context.

6. Presence of PJI is possible even if above criteria not met (based on clinical judgment).

Data from Osmon DR, Berbari EF, Berendt AR, et al. Diagnosis and Management of Prosthetic Joint Infection: Clinical Practice Guidelines by the Infectious Diseases Society of America. Clinical Infectious Diseases. 2012;56(1).

the Musculoskeletal Infection Society in 2011 (**Table 1**).[31,32] Within the Musculoskeletal Infection Society definition algorithm, 1 major criterion should be met, and, if not, then the minor criteria should be used to calculate a score. If the diagnosis is uncertain using the minor criteria, it is recommended to use the operative criteria to fulfill the definition of PJI.

Note that there are few randomized controlled trials analyzing the diagnosis and management of foot and ankle PJI, given the low incidence of these infections and numbers of procedures performed. As well, there are no guidelines outlining the standard of care for infection of internal and external fixation devices, so clinicians are often left to make decisions based on clinical experience (see **Box 1, Table 1**).

Microbiology

The IDSA guidelines outline *S aureus* as the most common cause of PJI (22%), followed by coagulase-negative staphylococci (19%), mixed infection (19%), beta-hemolytic streptococci (9%), aerobic gram-negative bacilli (8%), anaerobes (6%), and culture negative (12%).[33] In another cohort study of patients who had undergone primary or revision total ankle replacement, *Staphylococcus* species were found to be the cause of 70.6% of infections.[34]

Preoperative Diagnosis

Before operative intervention, a thorough history should be done to determine the type of foot or ankle prosthesis or implant, the date of insertion, the postoperative

Table 1		
Musculoskeletal Infection Society definition of prosthetic joint infection		
	Score	Decision
Major Criteria (At Least 1 of the Following)		
A sinus tract communicating with the prosthesis	NA	—
Two positive periprosthetic cultures with phenotypically identical organisms	NA	—
Minor Preoperative Criteria (Calculate the Score)		
Increased serum CRP level ($\geq$10 mg/L in acute PJI, $\geq$1 mg/L in chronic PJI) or D-dimer ($\geq$860 ng/mL)	2	• $\geq$6 Infected
Increased serum ESR ($\geq$30 mm/h in chronic PJI)	1	• 2–5 Possibly Infected
Increased synovial leukocyte count ($\geq$10,000 in acute PJI, $\geq$3000 in chronic PJI) or positive leukocyte esterase test strip	3	○ Use operative criteria to fulfill definition of PJI
Positive alpha-defensin ($\geq$1)	3	• 0–1 Not infected
Increased synovial PMN% ($\geq$90% in acute PJI, $\geq$80% in chronic PJI)	2	
Increased synovial CRP level ($\geq$6.9 mg/L)	1	
Intraoperative Diagnosis		
Preoperative score	—	$\geq$6 Infected
Positive histologic analysis of periprosthetic tissue	3	4–5 Inconclusive
Positive purulence	3	$\geq$3 Not infected
Single positive culture	2	

Abbreviations: CRP, C-reactive protein; ESR, erythrocyte sedimentation rate; NA, not applicable; PMN, polymorphonuclear neutrophils.
Chronic PJI is >90 d; acute PJI is <90 days.
Data from Parvizi J, Tan TL, Goswami K, et al. The 2018 Definition of Periprosthetic Hip and Knee Infection: An Evidence-Based and Validated Criteria. *The Journal of Arthroplasty.* 2018;33(5).

course, any wound healing problems, current microbiologic results, comorbid conditions, and other risk factors described earlier. A comprehensive examination of the foot and ankle should be done to inspect for erythema, edema, warmth, deformities, tenderness, range of motion, sinus tracts, and persistent wound drainage.

The onset of symptoms classifies these foot and ankle prosthetic infections into 3 categories: early-onset, delayed-onset, and late-onset PJI. Early-onset PJI occurs less than 3 months after surgery and is commonly caused by virulent pathogens acquired during surgery, such as S aureus, gram-negative rods, or anaerobes. Patients present with erythema, delayed wound healing, tenderness, and systemic symptoms. Delayed-onset PJI occurs 3 to 12 months after surgery, commonly caused by less virulent pathogens such as Propionibacterium acnes or coagulase-negative staphylococci, also acquired during implantation. The clinical course is often more indolent, with joint pain and a sinus tract, and generally without systemic symptoms. Late-onset PJI occurs greater than 12 months after surgery, usually secondary to hematogenous seeding with virulent organisms, and can present with sudden onset of pain in the setting of recent infection elsewhere. Notably, clinical symptoms are often not specific, and may be caused by aseptic mechanical complications.[11]

Erythrocyte sedimentation rate (ESR) and C-reactive protein (CRP) level should both be drawn but can be increased in noninfectious inflammatory conditions such as in the postoperative period, therefore trending these values may be of more utility. Optimal thresholds for prosthetic hip and knee infections for ESR are noted as 48.5 mm/h and 46.5 mm/h respectively, and for CRP are 13.5 mg/L and 23.5 mg/L, respectively.[35] There are limited data regarding optimal thresholds in foot and ankle infections. Blood cultures should also be done in patients who are systemically ill. New data show that interleukin 6 (IL-6) may play a role in diagnosis, with one study showing diagnostic odds ratios (ORs) of 314.7 for IL-6, 13.1 for CRP, 7.2 for ESR, and 4.4 for white blood cells.[36]

Plain radiographs with anteroposterior, lateral, and special hindfoot alignment views (Saltzman view)[37,38] of the foot and ankle should be done, but they lack sensitivity and specificity. Changes in position of prosthetic components, cement fractures, and periosteal reaction may be seen, but there is rarely clear evidence of infection such as a transcortical sinus tract.[35] Other imaging studies, such as leukocyte scan, are not routinely recommended and remain falsely abnormal in the postoperative period.[35] Computed tomography scans are limited by imaging artifact secondary to metallic implants, and MRI scans can only be done if implants are titanium or tantalum.[39,40]

Diagnostic arthrocentesis is recommended for suspected foot or ankle PJI if surgery is not planned, and antibiotics should be withheld for 2 weeks before collection of synovial fluid or periprosthetic tissue for culture. Synovial fluid analysis should include a total white blood cell count with differential, culture for aerobic and anaerobic organisms, and crystal analysis.[35] For patients with a TKA greater than 6 months from implantation without an underlying inflammatory joint, a threshold of greater than 65% neutrophils or a leukocyte count greater than 1700 cells/µL had a 97% sensitivity and 94% specificity for predicting PJI.[41] These cutoffs are notably much lower than in natural septic arthritis. In addition, sinus tract drainage should be cultured and correlated to other data because it may represent skin flora. The IDSA guidelines also suggests using leukocyte esterase strip to assist with diagnosis, which has a sensitivity and specificity of 93.3% and 77.0%, respectively, compared with positive cultures.[42]

Intraoperative Diagnosis

At the time of revision surgery, it is recommended to collect between 3 and 6 periprosthetic tissue specimens, and the explanted prosthesis if it has been removed, and to submit these for aerobic and anaerobic culture and histopathologic examination. Isolation of a single low-virulence pathogen, such as coagulase-negative *Staphylococcus*, in the absence of other criteria is not thought to represent a definite infection and should be evaluated in context, but isolation of a single virulent organism, such as *S aureus*, may represent a PJI. The optimal diagnostic threshold of polymorphonuclear (PMN) leukocytes per high-power field is uncertain; however, the IDSA shows that a threshold of 5 or more PMN leukocytes has a sensitivity of greater than 80% and a specificity of greater than 90%.[35] Gram stains are often negative, and false-negative cultures can occur when antibiotics have been given before collection, with fastidious or low number of organisms, or with delayed delivery to the microbiology laboratory, and so should be interpreted in the clinical context.[43] Submission for fungal or mycobacterial cultures is reserved for patients at high risk.

Delayed incubation of culture may assist with diagnosis, with one study showing that 26% of total patients with positive cultures had organisms detected after 7 days of incubation, predominantly *Propionibacterium* sp, *Corynebacterium* sp, and *Peptostreptococci*.[44] Various polymerase chain reaction (PCR) methods are being investigated for diagnosis of PJI and may have a role if antimicrobials have been given or for atypical organisms such as *Brucella* species. However, further investigation is necessary to understand the relationship between detection of bacterial DNA and clinical infection versus contamination.[45]

In addition, diagnosis can be complicated by the formation of a biofilm, a highly hydrated, extracellular matrix secreted by bacteria, which forms on the surface of prosthetic material. Inside the biofilm, bacteria enter a very slow growth phase, and in this state the bacteria are 1000 times more resistant to growth-dependent antimicrobials.[46] One method of increasing culture yield is to submit the explanted prosthesis for sonication and aerobic/anaerobic culture, which is thought to dislodge bacteria from the surface of the prosthesis.[26] Sensitivity has been shown to increase from 45% to 75%, comparing conventional tissue culture with sonication fluid, in patients who had received antimicrobial therapy within 14 days before surgery.[47]

SURGICAL MANAGEMENT

Current treatment stratagems are based on IDSA guidelines; nonetheless, data remain limited, with evidence for the following based on single-center noncomparative cohort studies and decision analysis.[35] Factors influencing surgical management include duration of syndrome, age of prosthesis, infecting pathogen, prosthesis stability, periprosthetic tissue quality, medical comorbidities, and patient preference.[35] The treatment strategies include debridement and retention, 1-stage or 2-stage exchange, permanent resection arthroplasty, arthrodesis, and amputation.

Kessler and colleagues[34] note that 61.8% with ankle PJI had surgery with retention of 1 or both components, 29.4% had both components replaced, and arthrodesis was done in 8.8%.[39] Another study, by Patton and colleagues,[6] showed a 21% amputation rate, with fusion rate of 10.3%. These procedures are often done by anterior incision, although the frequency of infection does not seem to be significantly different in the lateral versus anterior approach.[48] Ultimately, the IDSA guidelines recommend that management be left to the surgeons in consultation with infectious diseases, radiologists, and plastic surgery as necessary.

Debridement and Retention

Debridement and retention with or without polyethylene exchange is recommended if the patient has a well-fixed prosthesis, without a sinus tract, and is within 30 days of implantation or 21 days of onset of symptoms. Success rate is noted at 46% in one study of 14 TAA infections,[1] which is higher than for hip and knee PJI.[35] If these criteria are not met, the risk of relapse with this method is higher. Open arthrotomy is usually done, because arthroscopy seems to have worse outcomes.

One-stage Exchange

One-stage exchange (or direct exchange or revision procedure) is more commonly done in Europe, with success rates quoted as 80% to 90%. A 1-stage exchange involves:

- Excision of all prosthetic components and cement, send for culture and histopathology
- Debridement of devitalized bone and soft tissues
- Implantation of new prosthesis and usually antibiotic-impregnated cement

The indications for 1-stage exchange are:

- Healthy patients
- Adequate bone stock and soft tissue
- No sinus tract
- Easily treatable organisms such as *Streptococcus* species other than enterococci, MSSA, and non-*Pseudomonal* gram-negatives

Advantages include lower cost and fewer surgeries. There is a greater failure risk if bone grafting is required, because antibiotic-impregnated bone cement cannot be used. Of note, Kessler and colleagues[14,34] present 11 patients with ankle PJI who had undergone debridement and retention with severe soft tissue compromise as the single contraindication to implant retention. Ten of the 11 had relapse-free survival, indicating that grading criteria of soft tissue compromise may be too strict for PJI of ankle.[39]

Two-stage Exchange

Two-stage exchange (or staged exchange) is used more commonly in the United States, with a success rate reported at 87%. A 2-stage exchange involves:

- Removal of all infected prosthetic components, send for culture and histopathology
- Debridement of infected periprosthetic tissue and bone
- Insertion of local antimicrobial-impregnated cement or spacer
- Reimplantation of new prosthesis after infection is thought to be treated

Indications for a 2-stage exchange are:

- Medically able to undergo multiple surgeries
- With sinus tracts
- Difficult-to-treat organisms such as MRSA, enterococci, and *Candida*

Antimicrobial-impregnated static or articulating spacers are often used to manage dead space and deliver local antimicrobial therapy until a permanent prosthesis is placed. Both cemented and noncemented spacers are used and no specific cement material (metal alloys, ceramic materials, dense plastics) has been consistently shown to increase or decrease the rate of PJI.[35]

The time from resection arthroplasty to reimplantation varies from 2 weeks to several months, and, in the intermediate time, evaluation for residual infection is done with clinical examination, trending of inflammatory markers, and intraoperative inspection at time of reimplantation. One method often used is debridement, followed by 4 to 6 weeks of intravenous antibiotics, then an antibiotic-free period of 2 to 8 weeks before reimplantation. In selected circumstances, clinicians can retry a 2-stage exchange if the first attempt fails, although success rates are lower.[3]

Permanent Resection Arthroplasty

Permanent resection arthroplasty is resection of infected prosthesis without reimplantation. Indications for permanent resection arthroplasty include:

- Nonambulatory patients
- Limited bone stock
- Poor soft tissue coverage
- Infections secondary to highly resistant organisms with limited medical treatment
- Medical conditions precluding multiple major surgeries
- Patients with previously failed 2-stage exchange in whom risk of recurrent infection is deemed unacceptable

Eradication of infection occurs in 60% to 100% of cases, possibly with poorer outcomes because of selection bias.[35]

Amputation

Amputation is reserved for patients with the following indication:

- Necrotizing fasciitis not responding to debridement
- Severe bone loss
- Failure to achieve soft tissue coverage
- Failed attempt at resection arthroplasty
- Nonambulatory patients

Referral to a specialist center should be done before amputation.

Medical Management

Table 2 shows the medical treatment recommendations outlined by the IDSA guidelines. Addition of rifampin when treating prosthetic foot and ankle infections that have undergone debridement and retention or 1-stage exchange is required because of its ability penetrate the biofilm. Cure rates have been shown to be higher with combination of ciprofloxacin and rifampin for staphylococcal infection. Rifampin should not be used as monotherapy,[49] and use of rifampin early in the clinical course may increase the risk of rifampin-resistant staphylococcal selection pressure, so it is recommended to start after surgical treatment and initial antimicrobial therapy when bacterial load is less.[50,51] In addition, rifampin does not pass well through the membrane of gram-negative bacteria and is not recommended for gram-negative infections[52] (see **Table 2**).

The choice of initial intravenous antibiotics is outlined in **Table 3**, and causative organisms, pharmacodynamics and pharmacokinetic properties, tolerability, and susceptibilities should be considered,[53]

Intravenous antibiotics are commonly administered initially because of high bacterial load, with the risk of emergence of resistance being the highest during this

Table 2 Medical treatment recommendations		
	Staphylococcal Species	**Other Organisms**
Debridement and Retention	2–6 wk of pathogen-specific IV antibiotics + rifampin 300–450 mg PO q 12 h Followed by rifampin plus ciprofloxacin for total 3 mo for total hip/elbow, shoulder, ankle arthroplasty, and 6 mo for TKA • *Alterative to ciprofloxacin*: levofloxacin, cotrimoxazole, minocycline/doxycycline, first-generation cephalosporin, antistaphylococcal penicillin • *Alternatives to rifampin*: 4–6 wk of pathogen-specific IV antibiotic therapy	4–6 wk of pathogen-specific IV or highly bioavailable oral antimicrobial therapy
One-stage Exchange	Same as for debridement and retention	
Two-stage Exchange	4–6 wk of pathogen-specific IV/PO antimicrobial therapy (generally 6 wk for more virulent organisms such as *S aureus*)	
Amputation	Pathogen-specific antimicrobial therapy for 24–48 h after amputation if there is source control and patient is not septic. If there is residual infected bone or soft tissue, then use 4–6 wk of intravenous/oral antibiotics	

Abbreviations: IV, intravenous; PO, oral; q, every.
Data from Osmon DR, Berbari EF, Berendt AR, et al. Diagnosis and Management of Prosthetic Joint Infection: Clinical Practice Guidelines by the Infectious Diseases Society of America. *Clinical Infectious Diseases*. 2012;56(1).

period. Higher doses of antibiotics can be administered intravenously than by the oral route (ie, β-lactams).[54] However, the OVIVA (oral versus intravenous antibiotic) trial randomly assigned 506 patients to receive intravenous therapy and 509 patients to receive oral therapy no later than 7 days after surgical intervention, and intention-to-treat analysis showed noninferiority.[55] Regardless, it is important to use antibiotics that penetrate well into the bone. Data on bone level measurements of commonly used intravenous antibiotics are shown in **Table 4**, and bone levels of commonly used oral antibiotics are presented in **Table 5**.[54]

The guidelines do not outline management strategies for culture-negative PJI, which is estimated to be as many as 7% of patients with PJI.[32] Often clinicians are left treating with a broad-spectrum regimen that includes staphylococci, other gram-positive bacteria, and gram-negative bacilli, such as vancomycin or cefazolin plus ciprofloxacin.

Newer agents are available, such as ceftolozane/tazobactam and ceftazidime/avibactam, and may have utility for more resistant organisms, and the role of long-acting agents such as oritavancin and dalbavancin has yet to be delineated. Antibiotic toxicities should be monitored, including drug interactions with rifampin, a strong inducer of the cytochrome P450 isoenzyme, CYP3A4.

Chronic suppression

The IDSA panel was unable to come to a consensus on chronic suppression after debridement and retention or 1-stage exchange, whether to use in all or no

Table 3
Intravenous antibiotic treatment recommendations

Staphylococcal species	• If oxacillin susceptible:
	  ○ Nafcillin 1.5–2 g IV q 4–6 h, oxacillin or cefazolin 1–2 g IV q 8 h, or ceftriaxone 1–2 g IV q24 h
	• If oxacillin resistant:
	  ○ Vancomycin 15 mg/kg q 12 h
	• If oxacillin and vancomycin resistant or allergic/intolerant:
	  ○ Daptomycin 6 mg/kg IV q 24 h or linezolid 600 mg PO/IV q 12 h (few data published on combined treatment)

Enterococcus species	• Penicillin susceptible
	  ○ Penicillin G 20–24 million units IV q 24 h or ampicillin 12 g IV q 24 h (continuously or in 6 divided doses)
	• Penicillin resistant
	  ○ Vancomycin 15 mg/kg IV q 12 h
	• Alternative
	  ○ Linezolid 600 mg PO or IV q 12 h or daptomycin 6 mg IV q 24 h
	• Optional
	  ○ 4–6 wk aminoglycoside

Pseudomonas aeruginosa	• Cefepime 2 g IV q 12 h or meropenem 1 g IV q 8 h
	• Alternative
	  ○ Ciprofloxacin 750 mg PO q 12 h, or 400 mg IV q 12 h, or ceftazidime 2 g IV q 8 h
	• Optional
	  ○ 4–6 wk of aminoglycoside

Enterobacter species	• Cefepime 2 g IV q 12 h or ertapenem 1 g IV q 24 h • Alternative ○ Ciprofloxacin 750 mg PO q 12 h or 400 mg IV q 12 h
Enterobacteriaceae	• IV β-lactam based on susceptibilities or ciprofloxacin 750 mg PO q 12 h
Beta-hemolytic streptococci	• Penicillin G 20–24 million units IV q 24 h (continuously or in 6 divided doses) or ceftriaxone 2 g IV q 24 h • In case of allergy ○ Vancomycin 15 mg/kg IV q 12 h

P acnes	• Penicillin G 20–24 million units IV q 24 h (continuously or in 6 divided doses) or ceftriaxone 2 g IV q 24 h
	• Alternative
	  ○ Clindamycin 600–900 mg IV q 8 h or 300–450 mg PO q 8 h
	• In case of allergy
	  ○ Vancomycin 15 mg/kg IV q 12 h

Data from Osmon DR, Berbari EF, Berendt AR, et al. Diagnosis and Management of Prosthetic Joint Infection: Clinical Practice Guidelines by the Infectious Diseases Society of America. *Clinical Infectious Diseases.* 2012;56(1).

patients, or only those at high risk. Decisions are often made on an individual basis, weighing the risks and benefits of continuing an antibiotic for life. Duration of chronic suppression was examined in a 4-year study of 89 patients with PJI and debridement and retention, of whom 47.2% were free of infection 1 year after diagnosis. Suppressive antibiotics used for greater than 6 months was not associated with being free of infection (OR, 5.29; 95% confidence interval [CI], 0.74–37.8), but greater than 3 months was OR, 3.50; 95% CI, 1.30–9.43.[56] The IDSA recommendations for chronic oral antimicrobials for suppression are outlined in **Table 6**.

Table 4
Bone levels of intravenous antibiotics

Drug (Dose)	Patient No.	Serum Level, Mean (μg/mL)	Bone Level, Mean (μg/mL)	Ratio of Bone/Serum Levels (%)	Reference
Penicillin (2 g q 4 h)	1	5	Not detected	—	Smilack et al,[61] 1976
	1	0.5	Not detected		
	1	9.4	Not detected		
Methicillin (2 g q 4 h)	1	13.2	2.55	—	Ahmad,[58] 2010
	1	14.5	Not detected		
	1	15.5	1.05		
	1	50	2.25		
Oxacillin (2 g)	NA	NA	NA	10	Wewalka et al,[62] 1982
Oxacillin (1 g)	28	18.9	4 (cortical)	—	Warnke et al,[63] 1998
Flucloxacillin (2 g)	20	—	14.1	—	Bibbo & Goldberg,[60] 2004
Ampicillin (2 g)	20	NA	12	17	Warnke et al,[64] 1998
Ampicillin (1 g)	40	NA	20	33	
Sulbactam (1 g)	—	—	7	12	Wildfeuer et al,[65] 1997
Amoxicillin/clavulanate (2/0.2 g)	20	—	49.4/4.4 (cortex) and 34.6/3.04 (spongy layer) at 1 h	—	Bibbo & Goldberg,[60] 2004
Piperacillin (3 g)/tazobactam (0.375 g)	10	NA	NA	20/25	Incavo et al,[66] 1994
Piperacillin (4 g)/ tazobactam(0.5 g)	—	—	17.1/22.3	0.15/0.13	Bibbo & Goldberg,[60] 2004
Piperacillin (4 g)	NA	200	15	7.5	Bergogne-Berezin,[67] 2003
Piperacillin (2 g)	18	95	5	5	Kato & Morimoto,[68] 1984
Cephalothin (2 g q 4 h)	1	Not detected	Not detected	—	Ahmad,[58] 2010
	1	Not tested	Not detected		
	1	5.4	Not detected		
	1	13.2	Not detected		

(continued on next page)

Table 4
(continued)

Drug (Dose)	Patient No.	Serum Level, Mean (μg/mL)	Bone Level, Mean (μg/mL)	Ratio of Bone/ Serum Levels (%)	Reference
Cefazolin (1 g q 8 h)	1	>50	10.45	—	Ahmad,[58] 2010
	1	46	Not detected		
	1	Not tested	Not detected		
	1	31	Not detected		
Cefazolin (1 g)	35	80	10 (knee), 30 (hip)	13 (knee), 37 (hip)	Cunha et al,[69] 1984
Cefazolin (1 g)	20	45	8	18	Polk et al,[70] 1983
Cefazolin (1 g)	17	52	6	11.5	Williams et al,[71] 1983
Cefazolin (1 g)	48	NA	6	7.5	Schurman et al,[72] 1978
Cefazolin (2 g)	6	98	15	15	
Cefazolin (1–2 g)	16	25–216	3–10	<10	Fass,[73] 1978
Ceftriaxone (1 g)	13	104	20 ± 6	19	Lovering et al,[74] 2001
Ceftriaxone (2 g)	40	130	19 ± 7 (medullary) 6.5 ± 1.6 (cortical)	5	Soudry et al,[75] 1986
Ceftriaxone (2 g)	42	NA	17 ± 9 (medullary) 3 ± 0.7 (cortical)	NA	Scaglione et al,[76] 1997
Ceftazidime (2 g)	10	150	5 (ischemic legs)	3	Raymakers et al,[77] 1998
Ceftazidime (2 g)	10	—	3.4	—	Bibbo & Goldberg,[60] 2004
Ceftazidime (1 g)	43	NA	20	27	Leigh et al,[78] 1985
Cefepime (2 g)	10	73 ± 24 (cancellous)	74 ± 16 (cancellous) 68 ± 12 (cortical)	100 87	Breilh et al,[79] 2003
Cefepime (2 g)	10	—	99.8 (cancellous bone) and 67.6 (cortical bone)	—	Bibbo & Goldberg,[60] 2004
Imipenem (500 mg)	6	NA	6 (infected)	48	Handa et al,[80] 1997
Imipenem (500 mg)	10	13	2.6 (infected)	20	MacGregor et al,[81] 1986
Imipenem (1 g)	16	NA	4	16	Wittmann et al,[82] 1986
Meropenem (500 mg)	15	30	5.75	17	Sano et al,[83] 1993

Meropenem (500 mg)	—	—	15.4	—	Bibbo & Goldberg,[60] 2004
Ertapenem (1 g)	18	70.1, 10, 2.6 (at 1.6, 12.4, 23.8 h after administration)	15.2, 2.5, 0.6 (at 1.6, 12.4, 23.8 h after administration)	—	Bibbo & Goldberg,[60] 2004
Aztreonam (2 g)	18	—	16 ± 4.3	—	Bibbo & Goldberg,[60] 2004
Vancomycin (1 g)	14	22 (medullary) 22 (cortical) 16.8 (infected)	2.3 (medullary) 1.1 (cortical) 3.6 (infected)	10 5 21	Graziani et al,[84] 1998
Vancomycin (10 mg/kg q 8 h)	10	—	17.7 ± 5.7	—	Bibbo & Goldberg,[60] 2004
Vancomycin (15 mg/kg)	—	—	4.4 ± 7.6 (cancellous bone), 2.1 ± 1.5 (cortical bone)	—	Bibbo & Goldberg,[60] 2004
Daptomycin (6 mg/kg)	4	73	5	7	Traunmuller et al,[85] 2010
Daptomycin (8 mg/kg)	16	—	14.1 ± 11.9	—	Bibbo & Goldberg,[60] 2004
Daptomycin (6 mg/kg)	9	—	4.7	—	Bibbo & Goldberg,[60] 2004
Ciprofloxacin (200 mg)	20	NA	2 (medullary) 1.4 (cortical)	66 47	Meissner & Borner,[86] 1993
Ciprofloxacin (200 mg)	15	NA	0.1-0.9	3-30	Wacha et al,[87] 1990
Levofloxacin (500 mg)	9	8	6 (medullary) 3 (cortical)	75 38	Von Baum et al,[88] 2001
Levofloxacin (500 mg)	12	7.5	7.4 (medullary) 3.9 (cortical)	99 50	Rimmele et al,[89] 2004
Moxifloxacin (400 mg)	10	4.9	1.9 (medullary) 1.3 (cortical)	39 27	Malincarne et al,[90] 2006
Moxifloxacin (400 mg)	24	—	2.5	—	Bibbo & Goldberg,[60] 2004
Doxycycline (200 mg)	6	NA	2.6	86	Bystedt et al,[91] 1978
Doxycycline (200 mg)	25	NA	0.2	6	Dornbusch,[92] 1976
Doxycycline (200 mg)	25	—	1-1.1	—	Bibbo & Goldberg,[60] 2004

(continued on next page)

Table 4
(continued)

Drug (Dose)	Patient No.	Serum Level, Mean (μg/mL)	Bone Level, Mean (μg/mL)	Ratio of Bone/Serum Levels (%)	Reference
Doxycycline (200 mg)	34	6	0.13	2	Gnarpe et al,[93] 1976
Clindamycin (600 mg)	13	NA	5	67	Baird et al,[94] 1978
Clindamycin (300 mg)	27	7.33	2.63	40	Nicholas et al,[95] 1975
Clindamycin (600 mg)	23	8.5	3.8	45	Schurman et al,[96] 1975
Clindamycin (600 mg q 8 h)	1	12.5	9.26	—	Ahmad,[58] 2010
	1	10	7.33		
	1	3.4	Not detected		
Clindamycin (600 mg)	—	12.7 ± 4.5	3.4	—	Bibbo & Goldberg,[60] 2004
Metronidazole (500 mg)	16	NA	14	100	Hahn et al,[97] 1998
Metronidazole (1500 mg)	17	34	27	79	Bergan et al,[98] 1985
Rifampin (300 mg)	32	2	5 (1.4–8.8)	>100	Roth,[99] 1984
Fosfomycin (10 g once, then 5 g q 8 h)	19	NA	13.5 (uninfected)	NA	Meissner et al,[100] 1989
Fosfomycin (100 mg/kg)	9	377 ± 73	96 ± 15	25	Schintler et al,[101] 2009
Gentamicin (1.7 mg/kg q 8 h)	—	3.7	Not detected	—	Ahmad,[58] 2010
		Not tested	Not detected		
		4.8	3.66		
		7.1	Not detected		
Linezolid (600 mg)	13	—	3.9 ± 2.0	—	Bibbo & Goldberg,[60] 2004
Rifampin (600 mg)	32	—	2.7–16.7	—	Bibbo & Goldberg,[60] 2004
Dalbavancin (20 mg/kg)	—	—	13.4 (bone marrow), 4.2 (cortical bone)	—	Bibbo & Goldberg,[60] 2004
Oritavancin (20 mg/kg)	—	—	38.8 (tibia), 65.6 (bone matrix), 27 (bone marrow)	—	Bibbo & Goldberg,[60] 2004

Abbreviation: NA, not applicable.
Adapted from Spellberg B, Lipsky BA. Systemic Antibiotic Therapy for Chronic Osteomyelitis in Adults. *Clinical Infectious Diseases.* 2011;54(3):393-407.; with permission.

Table 5
Bone levels of oral antibiotics

Drug	Patient No	Serum Level, Mean and Range (μg/mL)	Bone Level, Mean and Range (μg/g)	Serum-Bone Ratio (%)	Reference
Ciprofloxacin					Fong et al,[102] 1986
500 mg	7	1.4, 0.4–2	0.4, 0.2–0.9	30	
750 mg	7	2.6, 0.9–4	0.7, 0.2–1.4	27	
500 mg	6	2, 0.9–3	0.7, 0.2–1.4	35	
750 mg	4	2.9, 1–6	1.4, 0.6–2.7	48	
Ciprofloxacin (750 mg)	—	4.3	—	27–48	
Ciprofloxacin (750 mg)	—	—	0.1–1.4	—	
			1.4 (cortical); 2 (medullary)		
Ciprofloxacin (750 mg)	—	—	1.4 with osteomyelitis, 1.6 without osteomyelitis	—	
Enoxacin (400 mg)	7	—	1.3	55	Fong et al,[103] 1988
Moxifloxacin (400 mg)	10	3.7	1.8 (medullary)	49	
			1.6 (cortical)	43	
Linezolid (600 mg)	13	NA	4	40	Kutscha-Lissberg et al,[104] 2003
Linezolid (600 mg)	12	NA	9	51	Lovering et al,[105] 2002
Linezolid (600 mg)	10	23	8.5	37	Rana et al,[106] 2002
Linezolid (600 mg)	—	11–21.1	—	40–50	
Linezolid (600 mg)	—	—	4–9	—	
TMP-SMX (1 DS tablet q 12 h)	14	7.4/143	3.7/1.9	50/15	Saux et al,[107] 1982
TMP-SMX (7–10 mg/kg/d TMP)	—	—	3.7	—	
TMP-SMX (160 mg)	—	1.72	—	50/15	
Fusidic acid (500 mg q 8 h)	15	NA	7.3, 1.7–14.9 infected bone	—	Hierholzer et al,[108] 1974

(continued on next page)

Table 5
(continued)

Drug	Patient No	Serum Level, Mean and Range (μg/mL)	Bone Level, Mean and Range (μg/g)	Serum-Bone Ratio (%)	Reference
Fusidic acid 500 mg q 8 h					
• For 5 d	9	27, 2–109	12, 1–40	44	
• For 6–10 d	15	45, 5–166	21, 2–75	47	
• For >10 d	14	27, 3–59	25, 3–79	93	
Fusidic acid 2 or 3 g/d	30	15–210	1.5–54	NA	Pahle,[109] 1969
Amoxicillin (500 mg)	—	5.5–7.5	—	3–31	Roberts,[110] 2014; Sendi and Zimmerli,[53] 2012; Clinical and Laboratory Standards Institute,[111] 2013 Lipsky et al,[112] 2012
Amoxicillin/clavulanate (875 mg)	—	2.2–11.6	—	3–30/1–14	
Cephalexin (500 mg)	—	12–30	—	18	
Cephalexin (1 g q 6 h)	13	—	2.5 d, 1; 5.9 d, 2	—	Bibbo and Goldberg,[60] 2004
Cefadroxil (250 mg)	52	0.2	5.1	—	
Cefpodoxime (400 mg)	—	4.5–7	—	15–30	
Clindamycin (600 mg)	—	7.5	—	40–67	
Clindamycin 450 mg q 6 h to 600 mg q 8 h	—	2.63–5	—	—	
Doxycycline (100 mg)	—	2.6	—	2–86	—
Doxycycline (100 mg)	—	—	0.13–2.6	—	
Doxycycline (200 mg)	6	—	4.9 ± 3.8	—	Bibbo and Goldberg,[60] 2004
Metronidazole (500 mg q 8 h)	—	—	14–27	—	
Rifampin (600 mg)	13	—	1.3 ± 1 (cortical bone) and 6.5 ± 1.3 (cancellous bone)	—	Bibbo and Goldberg,[60] 2004

Abbreviations: DS, double strength; TMP-SMX, trimethoprim-sulfamethoxazole.

Adapted from Spellberg B, Lipsky BA. Systemic Antibiotic Therapy for Chronic Osteomyelitis in Adults. *Clinical Infectious Diseases.* 2011;54(3):393–407.; with permission.

Table 6
Antimicrobials used for chronic oral antimicrobial suppression

Microorganism	Preferred Treatment	Alternative Treatment
Staphylococci, oxacillin susceptible	Cephalexin 500 mg PO q 8 h or q 6 h or cefadroxil 500 mg PO q 12 h	Dicloxacillin 500 mg PO q 8 h or q 6 h Clindamycin 300 mg PO q 6 h Amoxicillin-clavulanate 500 mg PO q 8 h
Staphylococci, oxacillin resistant	Cotrimoxazole 1 DS tablet PO q 12 h Minocycline or doxycycline 100 mg PO q 12 h	—
Beta-hemolytic streptococci	Penicillin V 500 mg PO q 12 h to q 6 h or amoxicillin 500 mg PO q 8 h	Cephalexin 500 mg PO q 8 h or q 6 h
Enterococcus species, penicillin susceptible	Penicillin V 500 mg PO q 12 h to q 6 h or amoxicillin 500 mg PO q 8 h	—
P aeruginosa	Ciprofloxacin 250–500 mg PO q 12 h	—
Enterobacteriaceae	Cotrimoxazole 1 DS tablet PO q 12 h	β-Lactam oral therapy based on in vitro susceptibilities
Propionibacterium species	Penicillin V 500 mg PO q 12 h to q 6 h or amoxicillin 500 mg PO q 8 h	Cephalexin 500 mg PO q 8 h or q 6 h Minocycline

Data from Osmon DR, Berbari EF, Berendt AR, et al. Diagnosis and Management of Prosthetic Joint Infection: Clinical Practice Guidelines by the Infectious Diseases Society of America. *Clinical Infectious Diseases.* 2012;56(1).

Prevention

The first measure of prevention of PJI is optimizing the patient's general health, and Marchant and colleagues[54] showed that patients with a higher hemoglobin A1c level had significantly higher incidence of PJI, with an OR of 2.31. Contraindications for ankle arthroplasty include active infection, peripheral vascular disease, deficient soft tissue, and Charcot neuroarthropathy.[57,58]

Surgical prophylaxis is imperative, with perioperative cefazolin used most frequently. Preoperative chlorhexidine may play a role, with one meta-analysis showing a 1.69% reduction of prosthetic knee infection.[59] Also, before arthroplasty a dental evaluation should be performed, and immunosuppressive therapy tapered if possible, although use of tumor necrosis factor alpha blockers in one study did not show an increased complication risk after elective foot and ankle surgery.[60] In addition, routine prophylaxis is not warranted for patients with foot or ankle arthroplasty before routine dental, urologic, or gastrointestinal procedures.

SUMMARY

Infection can be a devastating complication of surgically inserted prosthetic implants, such as joints for ankle, knee, and hip replacements, and intramedullary rods, plates, and pins for long bone trauma. Complications of infection include excessive antibiotic use, implant removal, reoperation, and potential amputation. Infections caused by colonized prosthetic implants are often difficult to predict, diagnose, and treat, because they form biofilms. It is important to recognize risk factors for PJI. Early recognition and treatment of PJI provide improved outcomes. Antibiotic selection is imperative for optimization of treatment, and surgical treatment strategies can include debridement and retention, 1-stage or 2-stage exchange, permanent resection arthroplasty, arthrodesis, and amputation.

REFERENCES

1. Lachman J, Ramos JA, Nunley J, et al. Outcomes of Acute hematogenous periprosthetic joint infection in total ankle arthroplasty treated with irrigation, debridement, and polyethylene exchange. Foot Ankle Int 2018;39(11):1266–71.
2. Yano MH, Klautau GB, da Silva CB, et al. Improved diagnosis of infection associated with osteosynthesis by use of sonication of fracture fixation implants. J Clin Microbiol 2014;52(12):4176–82.
3. Darouiche RO. Treatment of infections associated with surgical implants. N Engl J Med 2004;350(14):1422–9.
4. Gbejuade HO, Lovering AM, Webb JC. The role of microbial biofilms in prosthetic joint infections. A review. Acta Orthop 2015;86(2):147–58.
5. Althoff A, Cancienne JM, Cooper MT, et al. Patient-related risk factors for periprosthetic ankle joint infection: an analysis of 6977 total ankle arthroplasties. J Foot Ankle Surg 2018;57(2):269–72.
6. Patton D, Kiewiet N, Brage M. Infected total ankle arthroplasty. Foot Ankle Int 2015;36(6):626–34.
7. Myerson MS, Shariff R, Zonno AJ. The management of infection following total ankle replacement: demographics and treatment. Foot Ankle Int 2014;35(9): 855–62.
8. Kurtz SM, Lau E, Schmier J, et al. Infection burden for hip and knee arthroplasty in the United States. J Arthroplasty 2008;23(7):984–91.
9. Trampuz A, Zimmerli W. Diagnosis and treatment of infections associated with fracture- fixation devices. Injury 2006;37(Suppl 2):S59–66.
10. Zalavras CG, Patzakis MJ, Holtom PD, et al. Management of open fractures. Infect Dis Clin North Am 2005;19(4):915–29.
11. Kalore NV, Gioe TJ, Singh JA. Diagnosis and management of infected total knee arthroplasty. Open Orthop J 2011;5:86–91.
12. Hadeed MM, Evans CL, Werner BC, et al. Does external fixator pin site distance from definitive implant affect infection rate in pilon fractures? Injury 2019;50(2): 503–7.
13. Pfang BG, García-Cañete J, García-Lasheras J, et al. Orthopedic implant-associated infection by multidrug resistant enterobacteriaceae. J Clin Med 2019;8(2):220.
14. Kessler B, Sendi P, Graber P, et al. Risk factors for periprosthetic ankle joint infection: a case-control study. J Bone Joint Surg Am 2012;94(20):1871–6.
15. Kollrack YB, Moellenhoff G. Infected internal fixation after ankle fractures—a treatment path. J Foot Ankle Surg 2012;51(1):9–12.
16. Trampuz A, Widmer AF. Infections associated with orthopedic implants. Curr Opin Infect Dis 2006;19(4):349–56.
17. Park H, Kim H, Kim S, et al. Safety of temporary use of recycled autoclaved femoral components in infected total knee arthroplasty: confirming sterility using a sonication method. Clin Orthop Surg 2018;10(4):427.
18. Mody RM, Zapor M, Hartzell JD, et al. Infectious complications of damage control orthopedics in war trauma. J Trauma 2009;67(4):758–61.

19. Chen AF, Schreiber VM, Washington W, et al. What is the rate of methicillin-resistant Staphylococcus aureus and Gram-negative infections in open fractures? Clin Orthop Relat Res 2013;471(10):3135–40.

20. Romanó CL, Romanó D, Morelli I, et al. The concept of biofilm-related implant malfunction and "low-grade infection". Adv Exp Med Biol 2017;971:158–70.

21. Drago L, De Vecchi E. Microbiological diagnosis of implant-related infections: scientific evidence and cost/benefit analysis of routine antibiofilm processing. Adv Exp Med Biol 2016;971:51–67.

22. Gomez E, Cazanave C, Cunningham SA, et al. Prosthetic joint infection diagnosis using broad-range PCR of biofilms dislodged from knee and hip arthroplasty surfaces using sonication. J Clin Microbiol 2012;50(11):3501–8.

23. Cazanave C, Greenwood-Quaintance KE, Hanssen AD, et al. Rapid molecular microbiologic diagnosis of prosthetic joint infection. J Clin Microbiol 2013; 51(7):2280–7.

24. Portillo ME, Salvado M, Sorli L, et al. Multiplex PCR of sonication fluid accurately differentiates between prosthetic joint infection and aseptic failure. J Infect 2012;65(6):541–8.

25. Trampuz A, Piper KE, Jacobson MJ, et al. Sonication of removed hip and knee prostheses for diagnosis of infection. N Engl J Med 2007;357(7):654–63.

26. Berbari EF, Marculescu C, Sia I, et al. Culture- negative prosthetic joint infection. Clin Infect Dis 2007;45(9):1113–9.

27. Street TL, Sanderson ND, Atkins BL, et al. Molecular diagnosis of orthopedic-device-related infection directly from sonication fluid by metagenomic sequencing. J Clin Microbiol 2017;55(8):2334–47.

28. Esteban J, Gomez-Barrena E, Cordero J, et al. Evaluation of quantitative analysis of cultures from sonicated retrieved orthopedic implants in diagnosis of orthopedic infection. J Clin Microbiol 2008;46(2):488–92.

29. Esteban J, Alonso-Rodriguez N, del-Prado G, et al. PCR-hybridization after sonication improves diagnosis of implant- related infection. Acta Orthop 2012;83(3): 299–304.

30. Esteban J, Sandoval E, Cordero-Ampuero J, et al. Sonication of intramedullary nails: clinically-related infection and contamination. Open Orthop J 2012;6: 255–60.

31. Parvizi J, Zmistowski B, Berbari EF, et al. New definition for periprosthetic joint infection: from the workgroup of the musculoskeletal infection society. Clin Orthop Relat Res 2011;469(11):2992–4.

32. Parvizi J, Tan TL, Goswami K, et al. The 2018 definition of periprosthetic hip and knee infection: an evidence-based and validated criteria. J Arthroplasty 2018; 33(5):1309–14.e2.

33. Osmon DR, Berbari EF, Berendt AR, et al. Diagnosis and management of prosthetic joint infection: clinical practice guidelines by the infectious diseases Society of America. Clin Infect Dis 2012;56(1):e1–25.

34. Kessler B, Knupp M, Graber P, et al. The treatment and outcome of periprosthetic infection of the ankle. Bone Joint J 2014;96-B(6):772–7.

35. Honsawek S, Deepaisarnsakul B, Tanavalee A, et al. Relationship of serum IL-6, C-reactive protein, erythrocyte sedimentation rate, and knee skin temperature after total knee arthroplasty: a prospective study. Int Orthop 2011;35:31.

36. Berbari E, Mabry T, Tsaras G, et al. Inflammatory blood laboratory levels as markers of prosthetic joint infection. J Bone Joint Surg Am 2010;92(11):2102–9.

37. Saltzman CL, El-Khoury GY. The hindfoot alignment view. Foot Ankle Int 1995; 16(9):572–6.

38. Alrashidi Y, Galhoum AE, Wiewiorski M, et al. How to diagnose and treat infection in total ankle arthroplasty. Foot Ankle Clin 2017;22(2):405–23.

39. Kwee TC, Kwee RM, Alavi A. FDG-PET for diagnosing prosthetic joint infection: systematic review and metaanalysis. Eur J Nucl Med Mol Imaging 2008;35(11):2122–32.

40. Tande AJ, Patel R. Prosthetic joint infection. Clin Microbiol Rev 2014;27(2):302–45.

41. Bedair H, Ting N, Jacovides C, et al. The Mark Coventry Award: diagnosis of early postoperative TKA infection using synovial fluid analysis. Clin Orthop Relat Res 2011;469:34–40.

42. Wetters NG, Berend KR, Lombardi AV, et al. Leukocyte esterase reagent strips for the rapid diagnosis of periprosthetic joint infection. J Arthroplasty 2012;27(8):8–11.

43. Spangehl MJ, Younger AS, Masri BA, et al. Diagnosis of infection following total hip arthroplasty. Instr Course Lect 1998;47:285.

44. Schafer P, Fink B, Sandow D, et al. Prolonged bacterial culture to identify late periprosthetic joint infection: a promising strategy. Clin Infect Dis 2008;47(11):1403–9.

45. Hartley JC, Harris KA. Molecular techniques for diagnosing prosthetic joint infections. J Antimicrob Chemother 2014;69(suppl 1):i21–4.

46. Lopez D, Leach I, Moore E, et al. Management of the infected total hip arthroplasty. Indian J Orthop 2017;51(4):397.

47. Holinka J, Bauer L, Hirschl AM, et al. Sonication cultures of explanted components as an add-on test to routinely conducted microbiological diagnostics improve pathogen detection. J Orthop Res 2010;29(4):617–22.

48. Usuelli FG, Indino C, Maccario C, et al. Infections in primary total ankle replacement: anterior approach versus lateral transfibular approach. Foot Ankle Surg 2019;25(1):19–23.

49. Zimmerli W. Role of rifampin for treatment of orthopedic implant–related staphylococcal infections a randomized controlled trial. JAMA 1998;279(19):1537.

50. Spellberg B, Lipsky BA. Systemic antibiotic therapy for chronic osteomyelitis in adults. Clin Infect Dis 2011;54(3):393–407.

51. Achermann Y, Eigenmann K, Ledergerber B, et al. Factors associated with rifampin resistance in staphylococcal periprosthetic joint infections (PJI): a matched case–control study. Infection 2012;41(2):431–7.

52. Drapeau C, Grilli E, Petrosillo N. Rifampicin combined regimens for Gram-negative infections: data from the literature. Int J Antimicrob Agents 2010;35(1):39–44.

53. Sendi P, Zimmerli W. Antimicrobial treatment concepts for orthopaedic device-related infection. Clin Microbiol Infect 2012;18(12):1176–84.

54. Marchant MH Jr, Viens NA, Cook C, et al. The impact of glycemic control and diabetes mellitus on perioperative outcomes after total joint arthroplasty. J Bone Joint Surg Am 2009;91:1621–9.

55. Li H, Rombach I, Zambellas R, et al. Oral versus intravenous antibiotics for bone and joint infection. N Engl J Med 2019;380:425–36.

56. Keller SC, Cosgrove SE, Higgins Y, et al. Role of suppressive oral antibiotics in orthopedic hardware infections for those not undergoing two-stage replacement surgery. Open Forum Infect Dis 2016;3(4):ofw176.

57. Easley ME, Vertullo CJ, Urban WC, et al. Total ankle arthroplasty. J Am Acad Orthop Surg 2002;10:157–67.

58. Ahmad J. Total ankle arthroplasty as current treatment for ankle arthritis. Semin Arthroplasty 2010;21(4):247–52.
59. Wang Z, Zheng J, Zhao Y, et al. Preoperative bathing with chlorhexidine reduces the incidence of surgical site infections after total knee arthroplasty. Medicine (Baltimore) 2017;96(47):e8321.
60. Bibbo C, Goldberg JW. Infectious and healing complications after elective orthopaedic foot and ankle surgery during tumor necrosis factor-alpha inhibition therapy. Foot Ankle Int 2004;25(5):331–5.
61. Smilack JD, Flittie WH, Williams TW. Bone concentrations of antimicrobial agents after parenteral administration. Antimicrob Agents Chemother 1976;9(1):169–71.
62. Wewalka G, Endler M, Kraft A. Antibiotikakonzentrationen im Wundsekret und im Knochen bei gleichzeitiger Gabe von Mezlocillin und Oxacillin. Infection 1982;10(S3):S213–6.
63. Thabit AK, Fatani DF, Bamakhrama MS, et al. Antibiotic penetration into bone and joints: an updated review. Int J Infect Dis 2019;81:128–36.
64. Warnke JP, Wildfeuer A, Eibel G, et al. Pharmacokinetics of ampicillin/sulbactam in patients undergoing spinal microneurosurgical procedures. Int J Clin Pharmacol Ther 1998;6:253–7.
65. Wildfeuer A, Mallwitz J, Gotthardt H, et al. Pharmacokinetics of ampicillin, sulbactam and cefotiam in patients undergoing orthopedic surgery. Infection 1997;25:258–62.
66. Incavo SJ, Ronchetti PJ, Choi JH, et al. Penetration of piperacillin-tazobactam into cancellous and cortical bone tissues. Antimicrob Agents Chemother 1994;38:905–7.
67. Bergogne-Berezin E. Antibiotic tissue concentrations revisited in lungs. Crit Care Med 2003;31(8):2242–3.
68. Kato M, Morimoto R. Concentration of piperacillin in bone. Jpn J Antibiot 1984;37:279–84.
69. Cunha BA, Gossling HR, Pasternak HS, et al. Penetration of cephalosporins into bone. Infection 1984;12:80–4.
70. Polk R, Hume A, Kline BJ, et al. Penetration of moxalactam and cefazolin into bone following simultaneous bolus or infusion. Clin Orthop 1983;177:216–21.
71. Williams DN, Gustilo RB, Beverly R, et al. Bone and serum concentrations of five cephalosporin drugs. Relevance to prophylaxis and treatment in orthopedic surgery. Clin Orthop 1983;179:253–65.
72. Schurman DJ, Hirshman HP, Kajiyama G, et al. Cefazolin concentrations in bone and synovial fluid. J Bone Joint Surg Am 1978;60:359–62.
73. Fass RJ. Treatment of osteomyelitis and septic arthritis with cefazolin. Antimicrob Agents Chemother 1978;13:405–11.
74. Lovering AM, Walsh TR, Bannister GC, et al. The penetration of ceftriaxone and cefamandole into bone, fat and haematoma and relevance of serum protein binding to their penetration into bone. J Antimicrob Chemother 2001;47:483–6.
75. Soudry B, Sirot J, Lopitaux R, et al. Diffusion of ceftriaxone in human bone tissue. Pathol Biol (Paris) 1986;34:859–62.
76. Scaglione F, De Martini G, Peretto L, et al. Pharmacokinetic study of cefodizime and ceftriaxone in sera and bones of patients undergoing hip arthroplasty. Antimicrob Agents Chemother 1997;41:2292–4.
77. Raymakers JT, Schaper NC, van der Heyden JJ, et al. Penetration of ceftazidime into bone from severely ischaemic limbs. J Antimicrob Chemother 1998;42:543–5.

78. Leigh DA, Griggs J, Tighe CM, et al. Pharmacokinetic study of ceftazidime in bone and serum of patients undergoing hip and knee arthroplasty. J Antimicrob Chemother 1985;16:637–42.

79. Breilh D, Boselli E, Bel JC, et al. Diffusion of cefepime into cancellous and cortical bone tissue. J Chemother 2003;15:134–8.

80. Handa N, Kawakami T, Kitaoka K, et al. The clinical efficacy of imipenem/cilastatin sodium in orthopedic infections and drug levels in the bone tissue. Jpn J Antibiot 1997;50:622–7.

81. MacGregor RR, Gibson GA, Bland JA. Imipenem pharmacokinetics and body fluid concentrations in patients receiving high-dose treatment for serious infections. Antimicrob Agents Chemother 1986;29:188–92.

82. Wittmann DH, Kuipers TH, Fock R, et al. Bone concentrations of imipenem after a dose of imipenem/cilastatin. Infection 1986;14(Suppl 2):S130–7.

83. Sano T, Sakurai M, Dohi S, et al. Investigation of meropenem levels in the human bone marrow blood, bone, joint fluid and joint tissues. Jpn J Antibiot 1993;46:159–63.

84. Graziani AL, Lawson LA, Gibson GA, et al. Vancomycin concentrations in infected and noninfected human bone. Antimicrob Agents Chemother 1988;32:1320–2.

85. Traunmuller F, Schintler MV, Metzler J, et al. Soft tissue and bone penetration abilities of daptomycin in diabetic patients with bacterial foot infections. J Antimicrob Chemother 2010;65:1252–7.

86. Meissner A, Borner K. Concentration of ciprofloxacin in bone tissue. Aktuelle Traumatol 1993;23:80–4.

87. Wacha H, Wagner D, Schafer V, et al. Concentration of ciprofloxacin in bone tissue after single parenteral administration to patients older than 70 years. Infection 1990;18:173–6.

88. Von Baum H, Bottcher S, Abel R, et al. Tissue and serum concentrations of levofloxacin in orthopaedic patients. Int J Antimicrob Agents 2001;18:335–40.

89. Rimmele T, Boselli E, Breilh D, et al. Diffusion of levofloxacin into bone and synovial tissues. J Antimicrob Chemother 2004;53:533–5.

90. Malincarne L, Ghebregzabher M, Moretti MV, et al. Penetration of moxifloxacin into bone in patients undergoing total knee arthroplasty. J Antimicrob Chemother 2006;57:950–4.

91. Bystedt H, DAhlbäck A, Dornbusch K, et al. Concentrations of azidocillin, erythromycin, doxycycline and clindamycin in human mandibular bone. Int J Oral Surg 1978;7:442–9.

92. Dornbusch K. The detection of doxycycline activity in human bone. Scand J Infect Dis Suppl 1976;9:47–53.

93. Gnarpe H, Dornbusch K, Hagg O. Doxycycline concentration levels in bone, soft tissue and serum after intravenous infusion of doxycycline: a clinical study. Scand J Infect Dis Suppl 1976;9:54–7.

94. Baird P, Hughes S, Sullivan M, et al. Penetration into bone and tissues of clindamycin phosphate. Postgrad Med J 1978;54:65–7.

95. Nicholas P, Meyers BR, Levy RN, et al. Concentration of clindamycin in human bone. Antimicrob Agents Chemother 1975;8:220–1.

96. Schurman DJ, Johnson BL Jr, Finerman G, et al. Antibiotic bone penetration: concentrations of methicillin and clindamycin phosphate in human bone taken during total hip replacement. Clin Orthop 1975;(111):142–6.

97. Hahn F, Borner K, Koeppe P. Concentration of metronidazole in bones. Aktuelle Traumatol 1988;18:84–6.

98. Bergan T, Solhaug JH, Soreide O, et al. Comparative pharmacokinetics of metronidazole and tinidazole and their tissue penetration. Scand J Gastroenterol 1985;20:945–50.

99. Roth B. Penetration of parenterally administered rifampicin into bone tissue. Chemotherapy 1984;30:358–65.

100. Meissner A, Haag R, Rahmanzadeh R. Adjuvant fosfomycin medication in chronic osteomyelitis. Infection 1989;17:146–51.

101. Schintler MV, Traunmuller F, Metzler J, et al. High fosfomycin concentrations in bone and peripheral soft tissue in diabetic patients presenting with bacterial foot infection. J Antimicrob Chemother 2009;64:574–8.

102. Fong IW, Ledbetter WH, Vandenbroucke AC, et al. Ciprofloxacin concentrations in bone and muscle after oral dosing. Antimicrob Agents Chemother 1986;29:405–8.

103. Fong IW, Rittenhouse BR, Simbul M, et al. Bone penetration of enoxacin in patients with and without osteomyelitis. Antimicrob Agents Chemother 1988;32:834–7.

104. Kutscha-Lissberg F, Hebler U, Muhr G, et al. Linezolid penetration into bone and joint tissues infected with methicillin-resistant staphylococci. Antimicrob Agents Chemother 2003;47:3964–6.

105. Lovering AM, Zhang J, Bannister GC, et al. Penetration of linezolid into bone, fat, muscle and haematoma of patients undergoing routine hip replacement. J Antimicrob Chemother 2002;50:73–7.

106. Rana B, Butcher I, Grigoris P, et al. Linezolid penetration into osteo-articular tissues. J Antimicrob Chemother 2002;50:747–50.

107. Saux MC, Le Rebeller A, Leng B, et al. Bone diffusion of trimethoprim and sulfamethoxazole high pressure liquid chromatography (HPLC) (author's transl). Pathol Biol (Paris) 1982;30:385–8.

108. Hierholzer G, Rehn J, Knothe H, et al. Antibiotic therapy of chronic post-traumatic osteomyelitis. J Bone Joint Surg Br 1974;6-B:721–9.

109. Pahle JA. Experiences with fucidin in the treatment of osteomyelitis. Acta Orthop Scand 1969;40:675.

110. Roberts K. Oral antibiotics for the treatment of Adult Osteomyelitis: a tough pill to swallow. 2014. Available at: http://sites.utexas.edu/pharmacotherapy-rounds/files/2015/09/roberts09-26-14.pdf. Accessed January 3, 2019.

111. Clinical and Laboratory Standards Institute. Performance standards for antimicrobial susceptibility testing; twenty-third informational supplement. Clinical and Laboratory Standards Institute document M100-S23 2013. Available at: https://www.researchgate.net/file.PostFileLoader.html?id=55d77c2f614325f5d38b461b&assetKey=AS:273836702928896@1442299165694. Accessed March 1, 2019.

112. Lipsky B, Berendt A, Cornia P, et al. 2012 Infectious Diseases Society of America clinical practice guideline for the diagnosis and treatment of diabetic foot infections. Clin Infect Dis 2012;54(12):e132–73.

Lesser Digit Implants

Roya Mirmiran, DPM, FACFAS[a],*, Melissa Younger, DPM, AACFAS[b]

KEYWORDS

- Hammertoe • Surgery • Implant • Resorbable • Allograft

KEY POINTS

- There are several implant options in hammertoe surgery.
- One should be able to recognize the risks and benefits of available implants for hammertoe deformity.
- One should be able to appreciate improvements in technology while analyzing the cost-benefit of technology use.

INTRODUCTION

Lesser digit deformities are common pathologies treated by foot and ankle specialists. There are many contributing factors that result in lesser digit deformities at the proximal or distal interphalangeal joints. Overpowering forces such as flexor stabilization, flexor substitution, and extensor substitution have widely been cited as major contributing factors to digital contracture. Biomechanical advantages such as flexor stabilization, most commonly seen in pes planus foot deformity, is credited with being most common.[1–4] In addition, biomechanical alignment of the foot such as presence of cavus feet, a long second metatarsal, short first metatarsal, and hallux abductovalgus have been known to have great impact on development of hammertoe deformities. Factors such as aging, genetics, neurologic disorders, trauma with or without plantar plate injury, and soft tissue-occupying masses (ie tumors) have also been identified as possible etiologies.

As the deformity to the lesser digits worsens with time and the joints become less reducible, the treatment of the deformity becomes more challenging. Once nonsurgical interventions have been exhausted and symptom recovery has failed, surgical intervention may become necessary. The surgical treatment of a digit deformity can range from a simple flexor tenotomy to a rigid fixation of the interphalangeal joints or arthrodesis depending on how rigid the deformity has become. For a rigid digital deformity, an end-to-end arthrodesis is the common procedure, although other techniques such as a chevron or peg-and-hole arthrodesis are also described in literature. Limited surgical options exist to correct a hammertoe deformity exist, but the techniques used to

Disclosure Statement: The authors have nothing to disclose.
[a] Sutter Medical Group, 2725 Capitol Avenue, Sacramento, CA 95628, USA; [b] Independence Foot and Ankle Associates, LLC, 1401 North 5th Street, Perkasie, PA 18944, USA
* Corresponding author.
E-mail address: roya.mirmiran@aol.com

approach and stabilize the digit may vary. At times, additional procedures may be needed if there is added instability and/or deformity at the metatarsophalangeal joint (MTPJ). The traditional fixation device used to stabilize a lesser digit hammertoe correction is a smooth Kirschner wire (K-wire). This technique was first introduced in 1940 by Taylor.[5] Having said that, over the last 35 years, there has been many new devices introduced into the market to help with improving outcomes for a hammertoe correction. The goal of this article is to focus on advancements in technology as they relate to fixation devices used to achieve stability of the lesser digits at the proximal interphalangeal joint.

There are more than 60 intramedullary fixation devices available for use in hammertoe surgery. Although they all share the same common goal in providing stability and compression at the site of the arthrodesis, there are differences in strength and mechanical properties that may impact the overall structure and use. Properties of fixation devices include resorbable or nonresorbable material, single-component or multicomponent, dynamic versus static compression, and synthetic/metallic or allograft. This article focuses on use of 3 major subsets of implants:

Nonresorbable (K-wire, interosseous loop wire, single component, dual component, screws [solid or cannulated])
Resorbable
Allograft

The risks and benefits in use of traditional K-wire will be discussed before exploring the properties and advantages/disadvantages of non-K-wire implants.

NONRESORBABLE IMPLANTS
K-Wire Fixation

The traditional fixation device used to stabilize a lesser digit hammertoe correction is a smooth Kirschner wire (K-wire). Surgeons have utilized various sizes of K-wires from 0.035 to 0.062 inches wide to stabilize the digits. For ease of removal, a nonthreaded K-wire is frequently used. Although using a K-wire to correct hammertoe deformity is not a mandate, literature has shown better outcome and less recurrence k-wire stabilization. In a study of 54 patients with a 10-year follow-up, Holinka and colleagues[6] reported significantly less risk for recurrent deformity when the second digit was temporarily fixated with a K-wire versus a strapping dressing. Although substantial pain reduction was noted in both groups, the authors did not find a statistically significant difference in degrees of pain reduction after surgery in the 2 groups.[6] Stabilizing a hammertoe deformity is more of a concern, especially if there is an attempt for achieving arthrodesis at the lesser toe proximal interphalangeal joint (PIPJ) and/or if there is associated pathology, specifically at the second metatarsophalangeal joint (MTPJ).

K-wires can provide adequate stabilization across the joint. However, there is risk with rotational instability of a K-wire. Several articles present modified techniques in use of smooth K-wires for fixating a hammertoe correction. Recognizing that there is a risk for possible rotation and/or pin backing out, the authors suggest adding a second K-wire to provide rotational stability and increase compression across the fusion site.[7,8] A proposed technique is placing 2 smooth K-wires in a diverging fashion to provide the needed stability,[7] whereas another study simply proposes use of a 2-pin fixation across the proximal interphalangeal joints (PIPJ).[8] An alternative technique is use of a buried K-wire with aim at avoidance of K-wire exposure at the tip of the digit.[9–11] Despite use of buried K-wires, reported postoperative complications remain, including migration of the implant, nonunion, malunion, and infection.

An ease of revision, if needed, in comparison to other internal fixation methods is discussed.[10]

The length of time needed to maintain the K-wire in cases of PIPJ arthrodesis has also been studied. Klammer and colleagues[12] showed that 6 weeks of K-wire placement provides increased stability and lesser risk for recurrence. In their studies, 52 lesser toes were corrected using resectional arthroplasty of the PIPJ. A single K-wire was maintained for 3 or 6 weeks in 23 toes in each group. There were no statistically significant differences in AOFAS scores before or after surgery between the 2 groups. Recurrent malalignment was noted in 11 of 23 toes that had a K-wire for 3 weeks, compared with only 2 of 23 toes with a 6-week long K-wire placement. In a different study, prolonged K-wire fixation showed a more stable union with no increased risk for infection.[12] The weakness of this study, however, was the short 3-month follow-up time.

The use of K-wire fixation in hammertoe deformity correction has been in existence for many years, and such use is still highly practiced. Its use, however, has been associated with several risk factors. K-wires are known to migrate and result in premature removal and possible loss of stability. In addition, other complications such as pin tract infections and wire bending (**Fig. 1**) or breakage are also commonly reported.[13–15] Recurrence of deformity can still ensue despite 6 weeks of K-wire placement.[13–15] Zingas and colleagues[16] reported a 2.5% failure rate when a 0.045 inch K-wire was used in correction of a second digit hammertoe deformity. Pin tract infection has been reported in 18% of patients,[17] whereas a nonunion was evident in 20% of patients secondary to K-wire fixation.[18]

Recognizing the risks associated with use of K-wire fixation, there has been increased focus and enhanced effort in developing intramedullary implants for lesser digital surgery. There are several implants on the market, but only a few have a published comparative study.

Interosseous Loop Wire

Harris and colleagues[19] proposed a technique for internal fixation of an arthrodesis site using a 20- to 22-gauge monofilament wire. The wire can be used on its own or used as an augmentation to K-wire fixation. The monofilament wire is placed across the base of the intermediate phalanx and then routed in across the neck of the proximal phalanx to provide a box-type compression across the PIPJ. This technique requires simple instrumentation and is resistant to rotation or displacement.[19] As noted

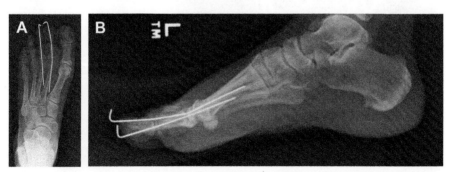

Fig. 1. Although the K-wire in the left third digit has remained straight, the K-wire in the left second digit is bent. The bend in K-wire can lead to additional postoperative complications such as infection or breakage, which then may result in early removal of the K-wire. (A) AP view and (B) lateral view of the same patient.

earlier, when utilizing this method, a K-wire can still be used across the MTPJ if needed for additional stability.

Single Component

One-piece digital implant fixation has been safely used in addressing hammertoe deformity. There are many types, but among all, the most interesting recent technology has been the use of memory nitinol devices (**Fig. 2**). Nitinol is a lightweight alloy that can return to its original shape after it is deformed. For instance, the implant can be maintained deformed frozen and when placed in the body, can return to its original shape. As such, this implant can provide compression and stability across the joint. The use of a 1-piece memory Nitinol intramedullary fixation device has been compared with the use of buried K-wires in several studies.[20–23] A retrospective study[20] of 118 digits showed no statistically significant differences in rates of nonunion or malunion or need for revision surgery between the 2 groups. Osseous union was reported in 68.9% of patients with this implant in comparison to 82.1% in patients with buried K-wires. Implant failure, however, occurred in 20.7% of patients

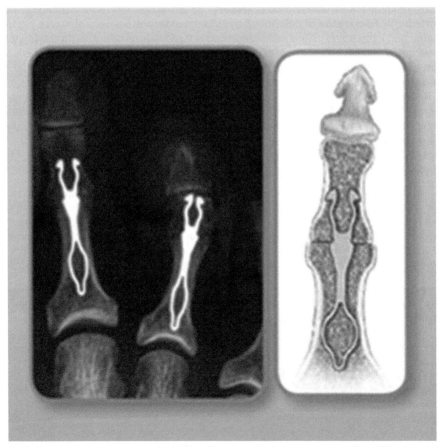

Fig. 2. One of the newer technologies involves use of a 1-piece memory Nitinol intramedullary fixation device. The memory Nitinol implant fixation is reported to outperform use of traditional K-wire in some of the studies. (Image reprinted with permission from Stryker Corporation. © Stryker Corporation. All rights reserved.)

with memory Nitinol implant and 7.1% of patients with K-wires.[20] Not all patients with complications were symptomatic; therefore, need for revision surgery was not significantly different between the 2 groups. In a smaller retrospective study, 28 patients were followed for 6 months after hammertoe correction using a K-wire or memory Nitinol implant. The memory Nitinol implant fixation was reported to outperform the K-wire stabilization.[21] A prospective study of 60 digital surgeries using the memory Nitinol implant showed an 85% rate of union with only 1 digital implant failure caused by dislocation of the device.[22] There were no cases of infection, and 86% of the patients reported no pain after surgery.[22] In a different study of 42 rigid hammertoe deformities, the effectiveness of a memory Nitinol device was studied,[24] and patients were followed for 1 year. The authors noted 81% osseous union among their patients, with 1 patient developing a minor digital rotational deformity. Sandhu and colleagues[25] retrospectively reported on the use of this implant in 35 patients (65 implants). A 93.8% arthrodesis rate was reported. There were complications in 4 toes. One complication resulted in an asymptomatic nonunion; 2 complications were due to hardware failure, and there was 1 implant displacement. No complications required revision surgery. The authors followed these patients for a mean of 27 months.[25] The use of this implant was further studied in a small population of patients (30 toes) with neuropathy.[26] The authors noted a stable nonunion in 7% of patients, with remainder of patients achieving successful fusion. There were other reported complications among this group, as 23% of patients noted to have a DIPJ contracture after implant placement with 13% suffering from a failed fixation.[26]

A different solid stainless steel-based (1-component) implant was studied and compared with K-wire in a retrospective analysis of 253 digits. A K-wire was used in 190 of the digits, with the remaining 63 digits having a 1-component device. The authors reported postoperative complication in 19% of digits (37 of 190) using a K-wire and 22.2% (14 of 63) using a 1-piece internal steel implant.[27] Malunion was seen in 7 of the digits fixated with a K-wire (3.7%) versus 4 patients (6.3%) in the intramedullary implant group. Superficial infection was reported in 4 cases with K-wire use, whereas no infection occurred in the internal stainless device group. There was no need for a revision surgery for either group.[27]

Dual Component

A multicenter randomized control trial of 91 patients compared the use of a dual-component stainless steel intramedullary implant against K-wire fixation.[28] There was no significant difference in incidence of complications between the 2 groups. The intramedullary device resulted in improved foot function and higher rate of fusion, as there was noted improved bone-on-bone apposition.[28]

In a retrospective study, use of a 2-component metal implant (in 95 toes) was compared with use of traditional K-wire (in 54 toes).[15] After following the patients for a year, the authors noted recurrent deformity in 9.5% of patients with K-wire fixation versus only 1 patient in the 2-component metal implant group. A late infection was seen in 3% of patients in the K-wire group. No infections were reported in patients receiving intramedullary implant. None of the patients in either group had a hardware failure. Revision surgery was performed in 5.3% of patients with K-wire fixation, whereas none of the patients in the intramedullary implant group required any additional surgery. Wound dehiscence (n = 1), complex regional pain syndrome (n = 1), and pulmonary embolism (n = 1) were seen in 3 separate patients. The authors concluded that use of an intramedullary implant is associated with better outcomes and fewer complications.[15]

Screw Fixation

Cannulated screws for fusion of the PIP joint, although rarely used, have been shown to provide successful results in union rate.[18,29] Caterini and colleagues[18] used cannulated screws to address 51 toes with hammertoe deformity. Complete arthrodesis was seen in 48 of the digits, with the remainder having asymptomatic nonunion. One screw was reported to be broken. Screw removal was necessary in 7 toes because of pain at the tip of the digit. A late infection was reported in 1 patient.[18] Based on available data, solid core screws may be used safely as well.

RESORBABLE IMPLANTS

Although the use of K-wire is not new to the science of toe surgery, inventors have developed a resorbable pin for use in foot and ankle surgery. Konkel and colleagues[30] studied use of absorbable intramedullary pin as a replacement for metallic K-wire fixation. Of course, use of a resorbable implant eliminated the need for pin management or removal.[30] The authors reported a 91% overall success rate,[30] with no incidences of an infection or toe swelling. Complete arthrodesis was noted in 73% of patients, with a fibrous union in 19%. The authors also noted 9 floating toes with another 8 digits having residual angulations among the 48 digits.[30] The authors confirmed the implant to be safe for use in hammertoe correction. Disadvantages for use of resorbable implant are possible lack of full resorption, late extrusion of the pin, and possible osteolysis of the bone around the implant seen on radiographs.[31] The absorbable pins are usually made of poly L-lactic acid (PLLA), polyglycolic acid (PGA), or combination of both and may not completely hydrolyze for at least 6 months after placement. Erythema and edema secondary to hydrolysis associated reactive processes can occur, although this is much less likely in implants with PLLA. The implant resorbs in time and is replaced by cancellous bone.

A retrospective study of 96 patients compared the use of a PLLA-based implant (27 toes), a Nitinol memory metal base (94 toes), and K-wire fixation (65 toes) with an average follow-up of 12 months.[32] The authors did not see any statistically significant differences in functional outcome or incidence of complications among the 3 groups. Although there were no significant differences in fusion rates, the patients with intermedullary fixation were noted to have a greater fusion rate. There was 10.6% implant breakage within 1 year in patients with Nitinol memory metal-based implant, which was significantly higher when compared with the other 2 means of fixation. All 3 implants were equally successful in achieving pain reduction.[32]

In a retrospective study of 297 patients with 377 1-piece polyetheretherketone (PEEK) implants, PIPJ arthrodesis was achieved at 1 year in 83% of patients. There was adequate deformity correction, with 94% patient satisfaction at 6 months.[33] The main issue with this implant was presence of continued moderate edema to the toe among 40% of patients at 6 months. After 1 year, 10% of patients continued to have moderate-to-severe digital edema.[33] Four (2.2%) of the implants had to be removed because of hyperextension at PIPJ and persistent pain. Varus positioning of the toe was noted in 2 patients after implant placement, with 3 intraoperative phalangeal fractures occurring at the time of implantation. Radiolucency around the implant was noted in 5% of the patients.[33] In another study by Harmer and colleagues,[34] a PEEK implant showed high patient satisfaction in 38 patients. However, there was postoperative incidence of 17.8% floating toes, 14.2% mallet toes, 17.8% metatarsalgias, and 10.7% transverse plane deformities in this patient population.[34]

ALLOGRAFT IMPLANTS

The use of allograft implants has been studied and compared with other implants. In a retrospective study of 96 patients, use of an allograft bone implant in 27 digits was compared with use of K-wires (65 digits) and memory Nitinol metal implant (94 digits). Overall satisfaction was 63% with K-wire, 68% with metal, and 87% with allograft.[32] Although the nature of postoperative complications varied among the patients with each implant, there was no statistically significant differences in functional outcome or postoperative complications. Wound dehiscence was highest among the patients with intramedullary implants (7.4% for each) when compared to K-wire fixation (4.5%). Recurrence rate and need for revision were higher in intramedullary implants, rather than the K-wire group. Implant breakage was only seen in patients with metal memory implant.[32]

Miller[35] performed PIP joint arthrodesis in 26 toes and found complete union in all but 1 patient. Fracture of the bone pin was found in 2 cases, but only 1 required revision surgery.[35] Similar union rates were also reported by Ford and colleagues[36] when using a cortical bone allograft pin to fixate hammertoe deformities in 30 toes.

IS NEW TECHNOLOGY BETTER THAN TRADITIONAL K-WIRE FIXATION?

Regardless of implant type, a digital surgery can always result in unwanted outcomes, and complications such as floppy, floating, and mallet toes in addition to deformity recurrence, nonunion, malunion, pin tract infection, implant breakage, and failure. The one thing common with deformity correction is that patient satisfaction and function are improved after surgery regardless of implant used. The K-wire use is inconvenient and concerning for both the surgeon and the patient. The current literature

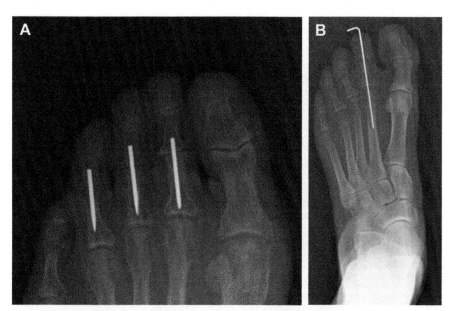

Fig. 3. Research has shown that patients prefer intramedullary fixation (*A*) over exposed K-wire fixation (*B*), although both devices provide similar pain relief. (*From* C. Clifford. Podiatry Today. What are the best options? Available at: https://www.podiatrytoday.com/hammertoe-fixation-and-cost-effectiveness-what-are-best-options; with permission.)

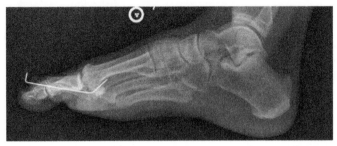

Fig. 4. One of the most common complications associated with K-wire fixation is hardware failure to include wire bending or breakage.

supports that patients consistently have higher satisfaction rates when intramedullary fixation is used, rather than K-wire (**Figs. 3–6**). Whether resorbable or nonresorbable, intramedullary implants share their own inherent risks and benefits. Disadvantages to use of implantable digital fixation are difficulty in inserting the device and even more challenges associated with explanting the implant if failure or pain emerges postoperatively. Need for revision is possible with any fixation methods. In a literature review by Guelfi,[10] the authors were able to analyze 9 studies comparing K-wire use against other advanced fixation implants. The authors reported no significant differences in patient satisfaction or total outcome when a K-wire was used versus other means of fixation. The arthrodesis rate among intramedullary implant in these studies ranged from 60% to 100%. Revision rates of 0% to 8.6% were reported for intramedullary implants. When a K-wire was used, revision rate was similar and up to 10%. Another concern with intramedullary fixation is the risk for breakage or failure of the implant. As such, the market has been and continues to focus on producing second-generation implants which reduce risk of hardware failure.

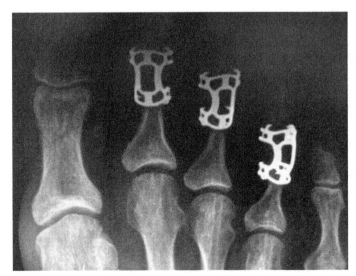

Fig. 5. Exotoe hammertoe fusion device. (*Courtesy of* M. Lee, DPM, FACFAS, Clive, IA, and Surgical Design Innovations, Park Ridge, IL.)

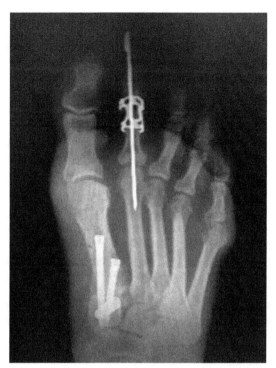

Fig. 6. Exotoe hammertoe fusion device with K-wire fixation across MTPJ. (*Courtesy of* M. Lee, DPM, FACFAS, Clive, IA, and Surgical Design Innovations, Park Ridge, IL.)

Although intramedullary implant is patient-friendly and appears to be more effective, the costs associated with such fixation may outweigh its potential benefits. Gained benefits are in exchange for significantly higher costs. A cost-benefit analysis should be considered prior to using any new implants.

SUMMARY

The K-wire for hammertoe deformity correction was first proposed and utilized in 1940 by Taylor,[5] and for almost 80 years it has remained the most commonly recognized and universally used implant for digital deformity correction. However, there have been exciting advances in technology over the last 35 years with the advent of intramedullary implants of various composition and architectural structures. The authors believe all categories of fixation method have the potential to achieve a satisfactory result, if used appropriately. Although research is still lacking when it comes to clinical trials, many of these devices stand out with strong case studies. Digital correction, similar to other surgical procedures, should include careful selection. One must place both the surgeon's experience and the patient's clinical picture and personal goals into consideration. Although authors of this article utilize K-wire fixation as the main course of treatment for hammertoe deformity correction, they recommend use of intramedullary fixation in cases of arthrodesis revision, in patients whom there is increased risk for pin tract infections, or for patients who might be a poor candidate for K-wire fixation.

There is continuous evolution, ongoing modifications, and advances in digital implants with aim at reducing postoperative complications in deformity correction.

Further evaluation and comparative studies are needed to determine the cost-effectiveness of the new devices in addition to outcomes. Despite much research being done in engineering, few randomized controlled trials exist in use and application of implantable devices.

REFERENCES

1. Myerson MS, Shereff MJ. The pathological anatomy of claw and hammer toes. J Bone Joint Surg Am 1989;71:45–9.
2. Thomas JL, Blitch EL, Chaney DM, et al. Clinical practice guideline: diagnosis and treatment of forefoot disorders. Section 1: digital deformities. J Foot Ankle Surg 2009;48:418.e1-9.
3. Shirzad K, Kiesau CD, DeOrio JK, et al. Lesser toes: review article. J Am Acad Orthop Surg 2011;19:505–14.
4. Zelen CM, Young NJ. Digital arthrodesis. Clin Podiatr Med Surg 2013;30:271–82.
5. Taylor RG. An operative procedure for the treatment of hammertoe and claw-toe. J Bone Joint Surg 1940;22:607–9.
6. Holinka J, Schuh R, Hofstaetter JG, et al. Temporary Kirschner wire transfixation versus strapping dressing after second MTP joint realignment surgery: a comparative study with ten-year follow-up. Foot Ankle Int 2013;34:984–9.
7. Hood CR, Blacklidge DK, Hoffman SM. Diverging dual intramedullary Kirschner wire technique for arthrodesis of the proximal interphalangeal joint in hammertoe correction. Foot Ankle Spec 2016;995:432–7.
8. Boffeli TJ, Thompson JC, Tabatt JA. Two-pin fixation of proximal interphalangeal joint fusion for hammertoe correction. J Foot Ankle Surg 2016;55:480–7.
9. Canales MB, Razzante MC, Ehredt DJ Jr, et al. A simple method of intramedullary fixation for proximal interphalangeal arthrodesis. J Foot Ankle Surg 2014;53:817–24.
10. Guelfi M, Pantalone A, Daniel JC, et al. Arthrodesis of proximal inter-phalangeal joint for hammertoe: intramedullary device options. J Orthop Traumatol 2015;16:269–73.
11. Creighton RE, Blustein SM. Buried Kirschner wire fixation in digital fusion. J Foot Ankle Surg 1995;34:567–70.
12. Klammer G, Baumann G, Moor BK, et al. Early complications and recurrence rates Kirschner wire transfixion in lesser toe surgery: a prospective randomized study. Foot Ankle Int 2012;33:105–12.
13. Kramer WC, Parman M, Marks RM. Hammertoe correction with k-wire fixation. Foot Ankle Int 2015;36:494–502.
14. Yassin M, Garti A, Heller E, et al. Hammertoe correction with K-wire fixation compared with percutaneous correction. Foot Ankle Spec 2017;10:421–7.
15. Richman SH, Siqueira MB, McCullough KA, et al. Correction of hammertoe deformity with novel intramedullary PIP fusion device versus K-wire fixation. Foot Ankle Int 2017;38:174–80.
16. Zingas C, Katcherian DA, Wu KK. Kirschner wire breakage after surgery of the lesser toes. Foot Ankle Int 1995;6:504–9.
17. Reece AT, Stone NH, Young AB. Toe fusion using Kirschner wire: a study of the postoperative infection rate and related problems. J R Coll Surg Edinb 1987;32:158–63.
18. Caterini R, Farsetti P, Tarantino U, et al. Arthrodesis of the toe joint with an intramedullary cannulated screw for correction of hammertoe deformity. Foot Ankle Int 2004;25:256–61.

19. Harris W 4th, Mote GA, Malay DS. Fixation of the proximal interphalangeal arthrodesis with the use of an interosseous loop of stainless-steel wire suture. J Foot Ankle Surg 2009;48:411–4.
20. Scholl A, McCarty J, Scholl D, et al. Smart toe® implant versus buried Kirschner wire for proximal interphalangeal joint arthrodesis: a comparative study. J Foot Ankle Surg 2013;52:580–3.
21. Angirasa AK, Barrett MJ, Silvester D. SmartToe® implant compared with Kirschner wire fixation for hammer digit corrective surgery: a review of 28 patients. J Foot Ankle Surg 2012;51:711–3.
22. Basile A, Albo F, Via AG. Intramedullary fixation system for the treatment of hammertoe deformity. J Foot Ankle Surg 2015;54:910–6.
23. Witt BL, Hyer CF. Treatment of hammertoe deformity using a one-piece intramedullary device: a case series. J Foot Ankle Surg 2012;51:450–6.
24. Catena F, Doty JF, Jastifer J, et al. Prospective study of hammertoe correction with an intramedullary implant. Foot Ankle Int 2014;35:319–25.
25. Sandhu JS, DeCarbo WT, Hofbauer MH. Digital arthrodesis with a one-piece memory nitinol intramedullary fixation: a retrospective review. Foot Ankle Spec 2013;6:364–6.
26. Roukis TS. A 1-piece shape-metal nitinol intramedullary internal fixation device for arthrodesis of the proximal interphalangeal joint in neuropathic patients with diabetes. Foot Ankle Spec 2009;2:130–4.
27. Scott RT, Hyer CF, Berlet GC. The PROTOE intramedullary hammertoe device: an alternative to Kirschner wires. Foot Ankle Spec 2013;6:214–6.
28. Jay RM, Malay DS, Landsman AS, et al. Dual-component intramedullary implant versus Kirschner wire for proximal interphalangeal joint fusion: a randomized controlled clinical trial. J Foot Ankle Surg 2016;55:697–708.
29. Lane GD. Lesser digital fusion with a cannulated screw. J Foot Ankle Surg 2005; 44:172–3.
30. Konkel KF, Menger AG, Retzlaff SA. Hammer toe correction using an absorbable intramedullary pin. Foot Ankle Int 2007;28:916–20.
31. Cicchinelli D. Hammertoe surgery and the trim-it drill pin. Foot Ankle Spec 2013; 6:296–302.
32. Obrador C, Losa-Iglesias M, Becerro-de-Bengoa-Vallejo R, et al. Comparative study of intramedullary hammertoe fixation. Foot Ankle Int 2018;39:415–25.
33. Averous C, Leider F, Rocher H, et al. Interphalangeal arthrodesis of the toe with a new radiolucent intramedullary implant (Toegrip). Foot Ankle Spec 2015;8:520–4.
34. Harmer JL, Wilkinson A, Maher AJ. A Midterm review of lesser toe arthrodesis with an intramedullary implant. Foot Ankle Spec 2017;10:458–64.
35. Miller SJ. Hammer toe correction by arthrodesis of the proximal interphalangeal joint using a cortical bone allograft pin. J Am Podiatr Med Assoc 2002;92:563–9.
36. Ford TC, Maurer LM, Myrick KW. Cortical bone pin fixation: a preliminary report on fixation of digital arthrodesis and distal chevron first metatarsal osteotomies. J Foot Ankle Surg 2002;41:23–9.

Charcot Neuroarthropathy Advances

Understanding Pathogenesis and Medical and Surgical Management

Georgeanne Botek, DPM[a],*, Samantha Figas, DPM[b],
Sai Narra, DPM[b]

KEYWORDS

- Charcot arthropathy • Charcot joint • Neuropathic osteoarthropathy
- Charcot neuroarthropathy • Charcot surgical treatment • Charcot pathogenesis
- Charcot advances • Charcot epidemiology

KEY POINTS

- Key advances have been made in investigating and reporting on Charcot neuroarthropathy epidemiologic pathways as well as the surgical approaches to managing the severe resultant deformities.
- The etiopathogenesis of active Charcot neuroarthropathy has evolved from a neurotraumatic and neurovascular theory to an osteoclast-osteoblast imbalance theory causing bone resorption, significant demineralization, and osteopenia.
- New genetic research is bringing us closer to unveiling the cause of Charcot neuroarthropathy with the ultimate goal of preventing the cascade of complex destruction.
- Treatment goals for an acute or quiescent Charcot process are to prevent skin ulceration and maintain or achieve a functional limb by creating a structurally stable, plantigrade foot and ankle.
- Current advancements in surgical techniques and fixation constructs include superconstructs spanning multiple joints and staged approaches for reconstruction combining external and internal fixation.

INTRODUCTION

In recent decades, 2 key advances have been made in investigating and reporting on Charcot neuroarthropathy: (1) research on and findings of the epidemiologic pathways, and (2) the surgical approach to managing the severe resultant deformities.

Disclosure Statement: The authors have nothing to disclose.
[a] Orthopedic Surgery, Cleveland Clinic, 9500 Euclid Avenue, Desk A40, Cleveland, OH 44195, USA; [b] Podiatry, Mercy Health Regional Medical Center, 3700 Kolbe Road, Lorain, OH 44053, USA
* Corresponding author.
E-mail address: botekg@ccf.org

Clin Podiatr Med Surg 36 (2019) 663–684
https://doi.org/10.1016/j.cpm.2019.07.002
0891-8422/19/© 2019 Elsevier Inc. All rights reserved.

Investigating the molecular, biochemical, and bone pathology of Charcot neuroarthropathy has propelled researchers in a way no one could have predicted 20 years ago. Transforming management from one of rest and watchful waiting to aggressively attempting to improve the quality of life for those afflicted by restoring a plantigrade foot are currently the 2 hallmark findings. Improved medical management and targeted therapies now lie on the horizon, which potentially could halt the cascading devastation that this syndrome has demonstrated, chiefly in the diabetic patient population with sensory neuropathy. The future is promising given the continued vigor and interest in understanding this limb-threatening complication. Continued research and education to increase awareness of the diagnosis of Charcot foot should be a goal of all physicians and surgeons who manage the advanced stages of Charcot neuroarthropathy. The average delay in diagnosis has been reported to be around 29 weeks[1] **(Fig. 1)**. Clearly, preventive medicine with early recognition is the most efficient, commonsense means to avoid severe deformity. Finding a confirming diagnostic marker, rather than relying on clinical suspicion or osseous changes seen in diagnostic imaging, could also lead to meaningful advancement toward better management and prevention of devastation.

Understanding the mechanism of such profound bony destruction, which is a hallmark sign of a foot ravished by Charcot neuroarthropathy, has long been an enigma since its first description more than 140 years ago. Modern concepts are exciting and better define the developmental pathway of Charcot neuroarthropathy, optimistically translating to earlier recognition and novel treatments beyond the historical gold standard of prolonged immobilization. Offloading gives the affected foot time to heal and arrests the progressive tissue damage and subsequent deformities. Offloading is maintained for as long as the foot demonstrates signs of inflammation, typically 3 to 12 months.[2–5] The sooner offloading is initiated in this acute process, the better the outcome.[6]

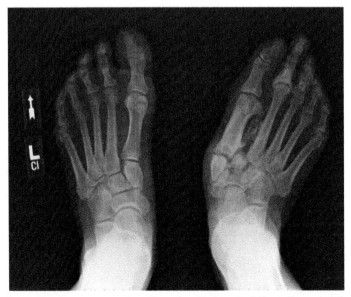

Fig. 1. Radiograph of anteroposterior view of a displaced midfoot Charcot deformity as a result of delayed diagnosis.

Charcot neuroarthropathy almost exclusively targets the foot and ankle.[7,8] Diabetes mellitus, with its complication of autonomic and peripheral sensory neuropathy, has become the predominant underlying conditional precursor to Charcot syndrome. The foot and ankle deformities that result from Charcot neuroarthropathy can dramatically affect lifestyle in a negative way, leading to disability and/or premature retirement from the workforce.[9] The effects of Charcot neuroarthropathy are devastating, reducing quality of life primarily because of decreased functional ambulation. Progressive Charcot leads to worsening deformity, which increases the risk of diabetic foot ulceration, infection, amputation, and even mortality.[10] Whereas the current prevalence is approximately 0.8% of the general diabetic patient population, this rate increases dramatically in the high-risk patient population to 13%.[11] Furthermore, the incidence of developing Charcot foot after receiving a kidney-pancreas transplant was reported to be 31% by Anthony and colleagues,[12] and 20% of persons with diabetes mellitus who received a kidney transplant developed Charcot neuroarthropathy an average of 7 years following transplantation.[12] Following kidney transplantation there is a 50% prevalence of osteoporosis and a 4-fold higher risk of fractures.[13] Pathophysiology may be attributed to abnormal bone metabolism related to parathyroid hormone, calcium, vitamin D levels, glucocorticoid use, and existing metabolic bone disease.[14]

ADVANCES IN UNDERSTANDING BONE DENSITY

In some respects, the bone changes visualized in Charcot neuroarthropathy can resemble those of osteoporosis, yet the interrelationships between diabetes, bone mineral density (BMD), and neuropathy are not fully understood.[15] In all cases of Charcot foot, 2 criteria are unequivocally present: inflammation and peripheral sensory neuropathy. How these 2 underlying conditions relate to bone pathology in Charcot neuroarthropathy is still not fully understood. Today, osteoclasts are generally accepted as responsible for the bone disorder observed in Charcot neuroarthropathy.[16] The etiopathogenesis of active Charcot neuroarthropathy has evolved from a neurotraumatic and neurovascular theory to an osteoclast-osteoblast imbalance theory causing bone resorption, significant demineralization, and osteopenia.[17–19] The 2 historic pathologic theories of the neurotraumatic and the neurovascular states do not fully explain Charcot neuroarthropathy on a molecular level.[20] The neurotraumatic theory states that unrecognized pain sensation leads to repetitive minor trauma in the pedal bones, resulting in damage to soft tissue and bone. This trauma can result from daily activities, infection, and surgery.[21] The neurovascular theory states that destruction of bone occurs secondarily to a hypervascular state occurring with loss of sympathetic function.[21] Blood flow has been shown to be 5 times greater in the neuropathic foot than in the sensate foot.[22] Autonomic neuropathy results in abnormal vascular reflexes with arteriovenous shunting and increased arterial perfusion, which has been shown in the neuropathic foot and the Charcot foot. However, the acute Charcot alone retains vasodilatory reflexes.[21,23] Edmonds and colleagues[24] found hyperemia commonly present in distal symmetric neuropathy, and concluded that patients are predisposed to excessive bone resorption and neuropathic fractures and that Charcot arthropathy can be caused by even minor stress.

Current evidence linking osteopenia directly with diabetic neuropathy is conflicting, however.[15] A recent meta-analysis did not find a significant relationship between diabetic neuropathy and poor peripheral bone health.[25] Specifically looking at BMD in Charcot neuroarthropathy, Petrova and colleagues[26] found a lower BMD in the non-Charcot foot of persons with type 1 diabetes mellitus but not in the unaffected side of those with type 2 diabetes mellitus, compared with healthy controls, yet both type 1 and type 2 affected Charcot feet had lower BMD than their respective contralateral unaffected sides. Sinacore and colleagues[27] and Jirkovská and colleagues[28] also found lowered BMD in Charcot feet, type 1 and type 2 combined, compared with their respective contralateral unaffected sides as well as controls. However, these studies have collectively been questioned since ultrasonic measures of bone density were used.[15] Although dual-energy X-ray absorptiometry (DXA) may currently be the preferred diagnostic examination, results from studies using DXA have been mixed.[29–31] Decreased bone density found in Charcot foot can also be secondary to immobilization itself and, as Christensen and colleagues[32,33] reported upon rescanning 9 years later, the BMD was no longer decreased. A more "regional osteoporosis" with increased osteoclast activity and unabated inflammatory response affecting bone quality may be a more accurate representation of acute Charcot neuroarthropathy.[19] Substantiating this idea, Jansen and colleagues[32] prospectively looked at BMD and markers of bone turnover and inflammation in 44 patients with diabetes, 24 of whom had a Charcot foot, between 2005 and 2007. The investigators concluded that patients with acute Charcot foot have elevated RANK-L/OPG ratios, with the levels decreasing over time to be comparable with patients without Charcot, and that no permanent effect of an acute Charcot foot on hip or bone density as measured by DXA of calcaneal and total hip BMD existed. Whether bone density or quality of bone is the same or similar among all persons with diabetes is another consideration. Regarding type 1 diabetes, studies show lower BMD levels and increased fracture risk.[34–36] In type 2 diabetes, however, the increased fracture risk that is seen may be more a question of quality of bone rather than bone mineral content, as BMD levels have actually been shown to be higher in persons with type 2 diabetes than in healthy controls.[37] Some investigators speculate that type 2 diabetes leads to a change in bone metabolism with poorer microarchitecture and altered bone turnover.[37–40] One study compared 23 patients' fracture patterns in Charcot neuroarthropathy with those of 23 dislocation-pattern Charcot cases and found an association with decreased peripheral BMD only in those with the fracture pattern[41] (**Fig. 2**). Comparing healthy bones with those of persons with diabetes and those with diabetic Charcot

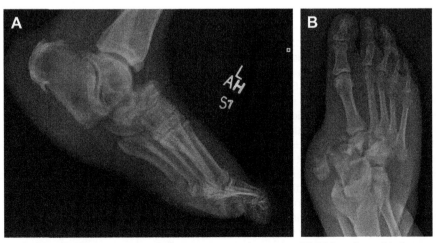

Fig. 2. (*A*) Dislocation pattern of Charcot neuroarthropathy. (*B*) Dislocation with fracture fragmentation in Charcot neuroarthropathy.

neuroarthropathy, La Fontaine and colleagues[42] found that, histologically, Charcot bones possessed inflammatory infiltrate of lymphocytes and eosinophils, as well as Howship lacunae and woven bone, suggesting inflammation and reduced bone density. Overall, the trabecular pattern was not completely unlike the non-Charcot diabetic foot bones that showed thinning trabeculae, reduced cellularity, and thickened tunica media of the vessels in the marrow spaces. The understanding of inflammation, bone changes, neuropathy, and the molecular pathway clearly is not complete with regard to Charcot pathogenesis.

BIOCHEMICAL PATHOGENESIS: INFLAMMATION

Jeffcoate theorized that, despite the hyperemia of distal symmetric neuropathy, exaggerated blood flow in the affected foot triggered by inflammatory stimulus is most important in the progression of Charcot arthropathy.[20,23,43] Modern theory has provided evidence supporting local inflammation as the cause of Charcot neuroarthropathy.[23] Local inflammation invariably occurs in the acute phase of the syndrome, and is the main symptom or sign that leads to the diagnosis, with or without radiographic evidence. The initial clinical presentation of an acute Charcot foot is a red, edematous foot with a temperature difference greater than 2°C compared with the contralateral site.[44] Inflammation as a potential aspect of pathogenesis was overlooked during the twentieth century because it was viewed simply as a result of continuing damage caused by loss of protective sensation in a well-perfused limb.[20] Jeffcoate and colleagues[20] hypothesized that an exaggerated inflammatory response to trauma—an insult that may or may not be recognized—is sufficient to trigger an inflammatory cascade through increased expression of proinflammatory cytokines, including tumor necrosis factor α (TNF-α) and interleukin (IL)-1β. This leads to increased expression of the nuclear transcription factor, nuclear factor (NF)-κB, which results in increased osteoclastogenesis. Osteoclasts cause progress to bone lysis, leading to further fracture, which potentiates the inflammatory process.

BIOCHEMICAL MARKERS LEADING TO A GENETIC BREAKTHROUGH

This dysfunctional osteoclastic activity has been deemed responsible for the bone changes seen in Charcot neuroarthropathy.[16,45,46] Osteoclasts, derived from monocytes and a central part of the osteolytic inflammation cascade, have become a predominant focus of concentration. Evidence suggests that increased systemic levels of biomarkers of bone turnover and inflammation exist in the acute Charcot foot.[33,47–51] A disproportionate osteoclast-to-osteoblast ratio and activity appear with a strong immune reactivity toward IL-1β, IL-6, and TNF-α.[15,52] Monocytes from patients with acute Charcot foot exhibit an inflammatory immune phenotype with increased production of proinflammatory cytokines such as TNF-α, IL-1β, and IL-6 compared with both healthy and diabetic controls.[53] Jeffcoate identified the RANK-L pathway as central to the pathogenesis of the Charcot foot, and an important piece in the puzzle of osteolysis, vascular calcification, and diabetic neuropathy in general.[31,54] Much research has focused on the receptor activator of NF-κB ligand, the RANK/RANK-L/OPG system. Osteoprotegerin (OPG) inhibits RANK-L actions, acting like a decoy receptor and the ratio it makes with RANK-L. A high ratio has been found in several reports of patients with Charcot foot, an expression of the current pro-osteoclastic and bone-related proinflammatory environment.[15,55,56] Mabilleau and colleagues[45] found monocytes from diabetic Charcot patients to differentiate into more active osteoclasts, especially when stimulated by RANK-L, and that OPG is insufficient to counteract it. Petrova and colleagues[57] have shown that osteoclasts from acute Charcot neuroarthropathy exhibited increased resorptive activity when exposed to RANK-L. By contrast, Jansen and colleagues[32] published data that showed an increased RANK-L/OPG ratio present only in the acute stage and not permanently elevated in persons with Charcot neuroarthropathy. Timing can thus make this biochemical marker elusive to isolate at various stages of Charcot neuroarthropathy. In 2018, Connors and colleagues[58] reported not finding a serum RANK-L/OPG ratio that was significantly different in patients with Charcot neuroarthropathy. Earlier in 2016, Bergamini and colleagues[59] also encountered conflicting data demonstrating no upregulation of RANK-L expression in circulating blood monocytes with acute Charcot.

The repetitive, unrecognized trauma secondary to neuropathy increases levels of the proinflammatory cytokines (IL-1β, IL-6, TNF-α), which could, in combination with a preinflammatory state, increase autoimmune reactivity and a profile of monocytes ready to transform into osteoclasts: cluster of differentiation 14 (CD14).[60] CD14-positive cells have the greatest propensity for monocytes for transforming into osteoclasts.[60] CD14-positive cells were found to increase, as were proinflammatory cytokine and TNF-α levels, in acute Charcot neuroarthropathy compared with diabetic and nondiabetic controls.[61]

Recently, one study was able to identify genetic markers and pathways that could play a role in the development of acute Charcot neuroarthropathy.[16] Charcot foot is characteristically identified today by exaggerated bone resorption, and increased numbers of osteoclasts may be attributable.[45–47] Osteoclasts, originating from monocytes, mostly CD14+, have the highest potential to differentiate.[62] Pasquier and colleagues[16] hypothesized that such circulating monocytes in patients with acute Charcot foot could be involved in the pathogenesis of the syndrome. These investigators studied blood samples from 18 patients with type 2 diabetes mellitus and acute Charcot, 18 patients with type 2 diabetes mellitus with neuropathy, and 18 patients with type 2 diabetes without neuropathy, and showed that methylation of circulating monocytes is involved in the pathogenesis of acute Charcot foot.[16] This type of research is transformative because it is one step closer to unveiling the cause of Charcot neuroarthropathy, with the ultimate goal of modulating or preventing the full-blown cascade of extreme inflammation and destruction.

Advances in Medical Treatments and Imaging

The etiopathogenesis of Charcot neuroarthropathy has shifted toward an osteoclast-osteoblast imbalance, although medical treatment studies logically first looked at the effectiveness of antiresorptive treatment with bisphosphonates. Bisphosphonates are antiresorptive drugs against osteoporosis, Paget disease, and other diseases with increased bone turnover.[63] Despite initial reports of the efficacy of bisphosphonates in active Charcot,[64,65] recent evidence does not support the use of bisphosphonates for active Charcot neuroarthropathy.[66,67] Perhaps safer than bisphosphonates, salmon calcitonin nasal spray daily with calcium supplementation has been studied in comparison with a control group that received only calcium supplementation.[68] Both groups were offloaded in removable cast walkers. The calcitonin nasal spray group did experience significant reduction of bone turnover during the 3-month follow-up. A benefit to calcitonin may be its direct impact on the RANK-L/OPG system with fewer complications.[69] After 3 months, patients who received daily salmon calcitonin nasal spray with calcium supplementation showed significant reduction of bone turnover compared with the offloaded group with calcium supplement alone.[69]

Yet another mechanism to consider in Charcot pathogenesis is one associated with hyperglycemia, neuropathy, and oxidative stress: the neuropeptides calcitonin gene-related peptide (CGRP) and nitric oxide (NO).[70] Neuropeptides likely are altered in the neuropathic foot and may contribute to bone turnover, but evidence is currently lacking. La Fontaine and colleagues[70] found in a small group of patients a significant decrease in endothelial NO synthase expression and a nonsignificant decrease in CGRP expression in the Charcot and non-Charcot neuropathic diabetic foot.

A single dose of RANK-L antibody treatment on acute Charcot neuroarthropathy, denosumab (Prolia), was studied in 11 patients in a comparison with 11 historical patients without the single injection of denosumab 60 mg subcutaneously.[71] Fracture resolution was significantly shorter compared with the usual-care group. Moreover, time to clinical cessation and malalignment in Chopart-Lisfranc joint at the end of total contact casting was also significantly shorter with denosumab.[71] A larger, randomized, and appropriately blinded trial will likely follow these early encouraging findings.

In January 2019, Rastogi and colleagues[19] reported on the use of teriparatide, or recombinant human parathyroid hormone, in 10 chronic Charcot cases, demonstrating a significant increase in foot bone remodeling with 20 µg administered subcutaneously daily in chronic Charcot neuroarthropathy when compared with 10 receiving a placebo for a 12-month period. Novel to this study was the utilization of fluorine (F)-PET/computed tomography (CT) imaging.[18] A dedicated PET/CT scanner was used at baseline and then again at 3 and 12 months. The anabolic agent increased BMD, which increased changes in the SUV_{max} (maximum standardized uptake value) in the teriparatide group compared with placebo at the region of Charcot neuroarthropathy, which was the midfoot in most cases.[19]

Advanced imaging with nuclear medicine, and now with images from PET/CT scans, have shown promising results, particularly with regard to recognizing early Charcot and that which is complicated by osteomyelitis.[72–75] PET has a distinct advantage over MRI in patients with metal implants. The addition of F-fluorodeoxyglucose (FDG) further enhances the diagnostic capability of PET.[76] Zhuang and colleagues[77] found FDG PET to be 100% sensitive and 87.5% specific for excluding chronic osteomyelitis. Similarly, Basu and colleagues[74] found a high negative predictive value in ruling out infection in diabetic patients with foot ulcers with FDG PET. Nevertheless, MRI remains the diagnostic test of choice in detecting early Charcot neuroarthropathy, with low signal intensity on both T1-weighted and T2-weighted images, juxta-articular bone marrow edema, and its familiarity and ease of access. In acute or stage 0 Charcot, MRI shows high diagnostic accuracy.[18,26,78] However, one cannot overlook the most important diagnostic study: the physical examination. A warm, red, edematous limb in a patient with sensory peripheral neuropathy and no open ulceration should be considered Charcot unless proven otherwise. After ruling out cellulitis, deep venous thrombosis, acute gout, and venous insufficiency, the diagnosis should become definitive with a high index of suspicion.

OTHER ADJUNCTIVE THERAPIES

Although electric bone growth stimulators have been used in acute Charcot and surgical cases, insufficient evidence exists to promote their use in the acute phase of Charcot with immobilization. Stimulators are more commonly used as adjuncts to postsurgical reconstruction.[79–81] Similarly, low-intensity ultrasonography for Charcot neuroarthropathy treatment has been described postsurgically.[82]

SURGICAL TREATMENTS AND ADVANCES

Despite promising biochemical, medicinal, and adjunctive therapeutic advancements in the treatment of Charcot neuroarthropathy, controversy remains over the most optimal treatment protocol for Charcot deformities. The use of goal-advanced surgical techniques in the correction of long-standing Charcot deformity is well documented in the literature.[83–86] Surgical intervention continues to become more prevalent with the advances in stronger, more anatomic fixation constructs as well as with better understanding of the technical aspects of surgical reconstruction of Charcot deformities. Kroin and colleagues[87] discussed the benefits of Charcot reconstruction on patients' quality of life. Their recent study mentioned poor quality of life in patients with Charcot neuroarthropathy, even in those undergoing conservative treatment.[87] They went on to demonstrate improved quality of life in patients who underwent successful Charcot foot reconstruction.[87] The gold standard of prolonged offloading and immobilization may be confined to the past as more clinicians seek to reclaim a functional foot through early medical prevention and surgical correction.

SURGICAL DECISION MAKING

Siddiqui and LaPorta, as well as Burns and Wukich,[83,84] presented indications for surgical intervention including unstable joints, nonhealing or infected ulcers with or without osteomyelitis, equinus deformities, and unbraceable deformities. The goal of any surgical intervention on a Charcot deformity is to create a plantigrade foot by restoring stability and alignment.[84,85] Reducing the deformity and restoring stability provides an ambulatory, braceable foot, which ultimately prevents ulceration and potential amputation.

Despite an increased understanding of the condition and the advancements in surgical techniques and implants, deformity correction remains controversial because of the multitude of comorbidities and high surgical risk associated with Charcot neuroarthropathy. Recently, several studies have evaluated prognostic indicators associated with complex Charcot reconstructions in this high-risk patient population. Elmarsafi and colleagues[88] performed a retrospective review and determined that postreconstruction nonunions, development of new Charcot joints, peripheral artery disease, renal disease, delayed postoperative healing, development of postoperative osteomyelitis, and elevated hemoglobin A_{1C} were common risk factors associated with major lower extremity amputation following Charcot reconstructive surgery. Rettedal and colleagues[89] developed a quick, usable prognostic scoring system to aid in surgical decision making of the Charcot foot. In their study, lower scores were associated with decreased ulcer recurrence and amputation following reconstruction.[89] Their prognostic score increased with advancing age, higher body mass index, presence of a wound or osteomyelitis, ankle involvement, active disease, and elevated hemoglobin A_{1C}.[89] Although surgical reconstruction of the Charcot foot is an important treatment modality in providing deformity correction and preventing ulcer recurrence, the risk of major limb amputation is high in this patient cohort and must be considered before undertaking any surgical intervention.

The timing of surgical management of a Charcot foot remains controversial, but often decision making has been assisted with the Eichenholtz classification system (**Table 1**). This 3-stage classification system described the radiographic progression of Charcot neuroarthropathy from osseous destruction and fragmentation, to resorption and coalescence, to sclerosis and joint arthrosis.[90] The additional prodromal stage 0, later added by Shibata and colleagues[91] in 1990 and further popularized by Yu and Hudson[92] in 2002, described the earliest manifestations of Charcot neuroarthropathy characterized by the clinical signs of inflammation that often precedes any radiographic changes. Surgical intervention during stage 0 or 1 has historically been contraindicated because of concerns for more wound-healing complications, hardware failure, and nonunions.[44,86] Stage 3 has historically been considered the most

Stage	Radiographic Findings	Clinical Findings
Stage 0 Inflammatory	• No evident radiographic findings	• Increased erythema and edema. Pedal temperature difference of 2°C–6°C compared with contralateral limb
Stage 1 Developmental	• Bony debris and loose osseous bodies • Subchondral bone fragmentation • Subluxation	• Erythema, edema, and warmth remain
Stage 2 Coalescence	• New bone formation • Absorption of bony debris • Fusion of joints	• Clinical signs of inflammation begin resolving
Stage 3 Remodeling	• Bony bridging • Ankylosis • Fx "healing"	• Loss of pedal architecture and deformity remains

Table 1
Eichenholz classification system for Charcot neuroarthropathy

Data from Papanas N, Maltezos E. Etiology, pathophysiology and classifications of the diabetic Charcot foot. Diabet Foot Ankle 2013;4:208–72; and Wukich DK, Sung W. Charcot arthropathy of the foot and ankle: modern concepts and management review. Journal of Diabetes and Its Complications 2009;23:409–26.

optimal time for surgical reconstruction because lessened risk exists for soft-tissue and osseous complications with the resolution of soft-tissue inflammation and osseous destruction.[93] Past treatment algorithms have recommended nonoperative immobilization during the acute phases, with surgical reconstruction reserved for the late chronic stages.[94]

With the improved understanding of Charcot pathogenesis and the advances in surgical techniques and constructs, surgical intervention is being integrated earlier in Charcot progression. Sella and Barrette[93] discussed earlier surgical intervention in stage 2 when the inflammatory signs are decreasing and the deformity remains reducible, as this prevents larger osseous resection and thus reduces the deformity that is often seen with reconstruction during stage 3. Simon and colleagues[95] followed suit evaluating arthrodesis in stage 1 Charcot, demonstrating promising results whereby all arthrodeses were successful, no patients developed short-term or long-term complications including reulceration, and all patients returned to their respective prior ambulation abilities.

Despite significant literature support, early surgical intervention remains controversial. With the recent advances in external fixation, a staged surgical approach has been discussed, because the risk of progressive deformities and potential limb loss remain without intervention. Lamm and colleagues[96] presented a 2-stage reconstruction involving deformity reduction with Taylor Spatial Frames followed by minimally invasive arthrodesis with beaming fixation. DiDomenico and colleagues[97] later described a variation on Lamm's staged approach involving deformity reduction with minimal osseous resection and external fixation followed by arthrodesis with aggressive osseous resection and various internal fixation devices.

PROCEDURE SELECTION

According to Siddiqui and LaPorta,[83] anatomic location of the Charcot deformity plays an important role in determining the success of treatment. However, no studies to date show predictability of outcomes based on location. A review by Elmarsafi and colleagues[88] contradicted this idea, presenting results showing that location of the joint collapse and the type of reconstruction performed bore no statistical significance to the risk of major lower extremity amputation. Location is, however, important in surgical planning. The anatomic location of the deformity will dictate not only the type of surgical intervention but also the implants used for fixation.

Depending on the deformity, tendon-lengthening procedures in conjunction with plantar exostectomies have good outcomes and are frequently used, the most common procedure being an Achilles tendon lengthening or gastrocnemius recession. Soft-tissue lengthening procedures in conjunction with an exostectomy have been shown to remove bony prominences and reduce plantar pressure, helping to prevent the probability of ulcer recurrence.[16] This combination is used when a severe contracture of the triceps surae is present, bringing the entire foot into an equinus position.[17] With increasing complexity and rigidity of the deformity, the worse prognosis is associated with exostectomies and soft-tissue balancing procedures alone. More complex Charcot foot deformities often involve arthrodesis to reduce the deformity and gain adequate stability.[84]

Soft-Tissue Balancing

Treatment strategies are often aimed at preventing ulceration and halting the acute phase of Charcot neuroarthropathy to avoid further degeneration and likelihood of ulcerations. Soft-tissue surgical intervention for Charcot neuroarthropathy is often a standard approach for balancing pedal pressure. Both tendo-Achilles lengthening (TAL) and gastrocnemius soleus recession (GSR) have shown evidence that they can heal Charcot foot ulcers as well as prevent their recurrence.[98,99] Procedure selection is made according to clinical findings of varying degrees of equinus. GSR is indicated for patients with mild equinus and history of Achilles tendinopathy. TAL is often performed in those with severe or spastic equinus, and a percutaneous approach can minimize wound complications in Charcot patients.[98]

Advantages of gastrocnemius recession include controlled lengthening and therefore prevention of a calcaneal gait, preservation of the Achilles tendon, and increased vascularity of the skin as well as the tendon for adequate healing potential.[98] The disadvantage is insufficient lengthening leading to ulcer recurrence.[98] Following a gastrocnemius recession equinus, the recurrence rate is 3-fold that of a TAL.[98]

TAL is indicated for moderate to severe equinus with a gastroc-soleus contracture. According to Maluf and colleagues,[100] there is an initial decrease in forefoot pressure after a TAL, but over the course of 8 months the plantarflexory muscles gain strength and forefoot and midfoot pressures resume. This is certainly something to consider and debate for the Charcot patient population, for whom we can conclude that TAL alone will not be sufficient treatment. An Achilles tenotomy is considered very aggressive and can be used in conjunction with a Charcot reconstruction. However, there is limited research into Achilles tenotomy alone for an equinus deformity, owing to its increased risk of both calcaneal gait and heel ulcerations.

Use of Early Gastrocnemius Soleus Recession for Charcot

Sanders and Frykberg[101] found that a preventable cause of the Charcot foot was due to an increase in plantarflexion forces combined with neuropathy with increased and repetitive mechanical stresses. It is believed that reduced range of motion, decreased tissue elasticity, and muscular imbalance, which is often seen with Charcot, along with equinus, leads to increasingly high forefoot pressures.[98,102] Greenhagen and colleagues[98] considered that GSR reduces forefoot pressure significantly and, therefore, could prevent Charcot development. This theory was tested when Laborde and colleagues[103,104] looked at patients with acute or chronic Charcot with and without ulceration and used a GSR, whereby they concluded that GSR could be used as an initial procedure for offloading the Charcot midfoot.[8] There is also current debate as to whether the use of GSR can decrease overall ulceration and prevent future amputations in the diabetic population.[104]

Muscle Flaps

First introduced by Ger in the 1960s, muscle flaps have gained popularity most recently. They are durable, have low donor site morbidity, and can be contoured to fill a dead space.[105] The most common intrinsic muscle used is the flexor digitorum brevis (FDB). The FDB is transected distally and raised to visualize the perforating vessels.[105] The proximal vessel remains and distal vessels are cauterized, then the muscle is rotated into the void of the ulcer and the donor site is closed primarily.[105] The biggest limitations of the muscle flap are the size of the actual muscle belly and the distance the muscle will reach.[106] Muscle flaps are an advancement in Charcot treatment because they are able to provide both coverage and vascularity to soft tissue and devitalized bone.[105,106]

Exostectomies

Exostectomy is a timeless procedure that has shown good results for Charcot patients without major deformities.[98–111] Often exostectomies are performed in conjunction with a soft-tissue balancing procedure to remove the prominence and decrease plantar pressures. According to Catanzariti and colleagues,[107] exostectomies are often the first line of surgical treatment typically performed after conservative management has failed. Exostectomies are preferred, and realignment arthrodesis procedures are used for further midfoot stability if the exostectomy fails.[110] Brodsky and Rouse[109] performed exostectomies in 12 of their Charcot patients, with 11 of the 12 healing their ulceration with no other breakdown over a 25-month follow-up period. Exostectomies are contraindicated in those with poor lower extremity arterial perfusion, acute infection, or unstable midfoot deformity, and in patients in stage 1 or 2 of the Charcot process.[107] Wukich and colleagues[112] found that with significant deformity at their lateral talar first metatarsal angle and calcaneal fifth metatarsal angle, Charcot patients are likely to ulcerate. Therefore, for those with significant deformity, exostectomies will not be an appropriate surgery. Currently there are 2 approaches, indirect and direct. The advantage of the indirect approach is the decreased risk of seeding infection into bone. Laurinaviciene and colleagues[110] performed a 19-person study using indirect approaches along the base of the exostosis (medial or lateral) to avoid the ulcer itself. If the exostosis was on the medial column, a full-thickness incision was made medially along the base of the exostosis.[110] Alternatively, the direct approach is used to remove the prominence through the ulceration and excise the ulcer. The ulcer can be primarily closed or heal by secondary intention based on the surgeon's preference. Regardless of approach, the prominence is removed with a saw or osteotome and removal is parallel to the weight-bearing surface.[107] It is known that ulcers on the lateral column have a higher complication rate than that of the medial column, and thus may require multiple procedures and exostectomies to properly heal.[107,110]

EXTERNAL FIXATION

Complex rigid or unstable deformities not amenable to exostectomies or soft-tissue balancing procedures often require more invasive procedures, including midfoot and rearfoot arthrodesis. Charcot foot reconstructions are often complicated by the compromised soft tissue and bone.[85,99] Many of these patients already have chronic ulcerations and osteomyelitis, as well as many comorbidities that decrease their healing potential. Arthrodesis with internal fixation is often contraindicated in these patients given the increased risk for recurrent infections, inadequate soft-tissue coverage over the hardware, and hardware failure resulting from compromised bone quality.[85,99,113] External fixation can be an alternative technique for patients for whom internal fixation is unsuitable or for a staged reconstruction approach.

External fixation allows for minimally invasive surgical intervention that can provide stability across several joints while avoiding potentially infected or compromised bone and damage to the soft-tissue envelope. Recent literature contains inconclusive data comparing internal and external fixation in the treatment of Charcot foot deformities.[113,114] Many improvements in external fixation devices have been developed in recent years, which has allowed this fixation method to gain popularity, especially in Charcot reconstruction.

The first form of external fixation was described by Hippocrates, whereby leather rings and wooden rods were used to splint tibial fractures.[115] Over the next 2000 years, external fixation developed into monolateral and circular devices.[115] Monolateral external fixation neutralizes deforming forces by providing relative stability to maintain reduction; it is therefore considered "flexible" and consequently more difficult to achieve absolute rigidity to achieve primary bone healing. Therefore, monolateral external fixation is considered temporary and is often used in a 2-stage reconstruction approach.

Over the years, monolateral external fixation has advanced to both uniplanar and biplanar frames.[115] Biplanar external fixation is more commonly used for Charcot reconstruction in the form of a Delta frame.[116] Over the years, components of Delta frames have been modified, transitioning from stainless-steel rods to radiolucent carbon fiber rods. Kowalski and colleagues[117] discussed not only their radiolucency but also the increased stiffness of carbon fiber rods compared with stainless steel. Their study found carbon fiber to be 15% stiffer than stainless steel, thus producing a better environment for primary bone healing by increasing construct rigidity.[117]

Circular external fixator frames are an alternative to Delta frames for Charcot foot reconstruction (**Fig. 3**). Ilizarov first developed this newer method of external fixation in the 1950s for the treatment of fracture nonunions in the lower leg.[118] This external

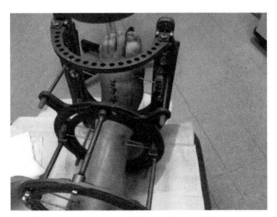

Fig. 3. Circular external fixation is considered biomechanically superior to other external fixation devices that can be used in staged or definitive Charcot reconstructions, as these constructs prevent angulation and rotation while still allowing axial compression.

fixation technique has since been adapted to assist with staged or definitive reconstruction of Charcot foot, as circular fixators are biomechanically superior to Delta frames in their prevention of angulation and rotation while still allowing axial compression to assist with the healing of arthrodesis sites.

Patients who benefit from external fixation are often those with histories of chronic ulcerations, osteomyelitis, and compromised soft-tissue envelope.[85,99,113] However, external fixators are not without their complications, whether using Delta or Ilizarov frames. Disadvantages of using external fixation include higher risk of neurovascular injury, infection caused by exposed hardware for long periods of time, and malunions or nonunions resulting from lack of compression through the frames compared with internal fixation.[118] Given these risks as well as the high learning curve associated with external fixation application, some surgeons prefer internal fixation as their method of choice.

INTERNAL FIXATION

Internal fixation using plates, screws, or intramedullary nail devices has been commonly described alongside external fixation in the treatment of Charcot deformity. Advantages of internal fixation include greater immobilization compared with external fixation by creating greater compression across arthrodesis sites, and buried fixation leading to decreased risk of hardware infections.

Throughout the literature, various methods of internal fixation have been described to assist with arthrodesis of damaged Charcot joints. Until recently, surgeons were concerned with the ability of internal fixation to span several joints while avoiding infected or essentially dead bone associated with the Charcot foot. In 2009, Sammarco[119] described the idea of a "superconstruct," whereby the internal fixation extends beyond the affected joints to gain adequate purchase in nonaffected bone. Sammarco described 4 basic principles of a superconstruct: (1) bone resection to correct deformity and decrease soft-tissue tension, (2) optimal position that maximizes mechanical function, (3) arthrodesis extending beyond affected joints to improve fixation, and (4) use of strongest hardware that can be tolerated by the soft-tissue envelope[119] (**Fig. 4**). Beaming and plating are 2 techniques used to create these internal

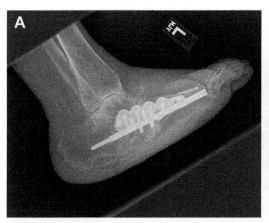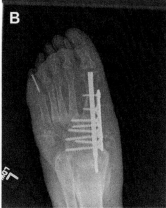

Fig. 4. (*A*) Lateral view of superconstruct Charcot reconstruction with intramedullary screw and plating of medial column. (*B*) Anteroposterior radiograph of superconstruct in Charcot reconstruction with intramedullary fixation and plate/screw construct.

fixation superconstructs for Charcot foot reconstructions. Pope and colleagues[120] presented a cadaveric study comparing beaming with plating and concluded that no notable differences exist between the 2 fixation techniques when used in Charcot reconstructions.

BEAMING

Beaming or intramedullary fixation allows for minimally invasive fixation across multiple joints without significant soft-tissue compromise. Beaming also provides stress shielding, both dorsal and plantar, which is often difficult with plating systems.[1] In Charcot foot reconstruction, beaming is typically performed using large-diameter, long-length solid screws. The importance of lateral column beaming was discussed by Grant and colleagues,[121] who found the prevalence of lateral column collapse following medial column beaming owing to the increased mechanical advantage of the tibialis posterior tendon causing inversion and lateral column overloading. Grant and colleagues[121] also discussed the importance of inclusion of the rear foot, specifically the subtalar joint, when beaming the medial and lateral columns to provide stability to the transverse arch. When the ankle is also involved in the Charcot deformity, intramedullary nails are often considered stronger constructions.[113] Wukich and colleagues[122] and Noonan and colleagues[123] discuss the use of longer nails than shorter nails to prevent varus or valgus toggling, which can lead to stress reaction at the proximal screw hole.

When using beams in the foot, optimal fixation is achieved by maximizing screw-to-bone purchase. Undersizing implants can cause construct failure, and oversizing can cause an iatrogenic fracture.[124] Disadvantages to beaming include lack of compression to facilitate arthrodesis and minimal to no frontal plane stability.[124]

PLATING

Bridge plating is a well-known fixation method in trauma settings, most commonly seen with comminuted fractures. However, with the popularization of anatomic locking plates in foot and ankle reconstruction, bridge-plating techniques have been adapted to assist with extended joint arthrodesis or superconstructs of Charcot foot reconstructions[119] (**Fig 5**). Advantages to using bridge-plating technique over intramedullary fixation include better visualization and preparation of affected joints, which allows for easier reduction of dislocations and deformities associated with Charcot

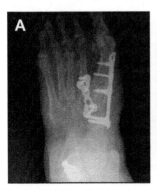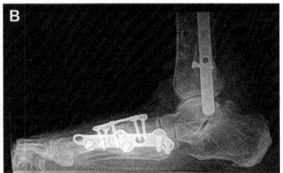

Fig. 5. (A) Extended joint arthrodesis with bridge plating in Charcot reconstruction. (B) Lateral view of plating in Charcot foot reconstruction.

foot.[125] Other key advantages of this technique are the increased compression to aid in arthrodesis, stability in the transverse plane, and the ease of application.[125]

Plating systems are not without disadvantages. Charcot patients are already at high risk of postoperative complications given their poor soft-tissue envelopes, inadequate bone stock, and decreased healing potential. Therefore, the use of expansive plating systems increases the risk of wound-healing complications, as locking plates require larger incisions for placement.[125] This could ultimately lead to exposed hardware, increasing the risk of postoperative infections. A patient's poor bone stock may also lead to a lack of purchase of the plates and screws, which could lead to malunions or nonunions.[125]

One type of plating technique for Charcot foot reconstruction is plantar plating. Fixation along the tension side of the foot counteracts the deforming forces exerted on the foot during weight bearing.[125] Garchar and colleagues[126] described a plantar plating technique that demonstrated a strong, sturdy construct allowing for earlier ambulation whereby their mean interval to ambulation was less than 12 weeks. However, extensive dissection is required to apply plantar plates throughout the midfoot, which can lead to wound-healing complications in the already compromised diabetic patient.[125]

Another type of plating technique for Charcot foot reconstruction is extended medial column plating. This allows for maximum construct stability with minimal soft-tissue dissection when compared with plantar plating.[119,126,127] Initially carried out with traditional nonlocking or buttressing plates, it has since evolved into the utilization of locking plate systems with the popularization of superconstruct principles.[119] Locking plates allow for stronger, more stable constructs when compared with traditional plating systems.[125,128] These newer plating systems often allow for variable-angle or polyaxial screws, which assists with joint-specific contouring that is not always amenable with traditional plating or beaming constructs.[125,129] Cullen and colleagues[129] demonstrated the enhanced stability of plating systems that allowed for polyaxial screw fixation. Charcot-indicated–specific plates, such as the SALVATION 3Di Plating System (Wright Medical Technology, Arlington, TN, USA), VA LCP Medial Column Fusion Plates (DePuy Synthes, Raynham, MA, USA), and VLP FOOT Column Fusion Plate (Smith and Nephew, Cordova, TN, USA) are becoming more popular with extended medial column arthrodesis, as the plating systems are anatomically contoured to span the talonavicular, naviculocuneiform, and first tarsometatarsal joints. They also allow both polyaxial nonlocking and locking screw fixation to aid in stability and compression at the arthrodesis sites.[125]

SUMMARY

Charcot neuroarthropathy is a complex syndrome of microfractures, dislocations, and soft-tissue changes affecting predominantly the foot and ankle in the neuropathic extremity, chiefly affecting persons with diabetes mellitus. Making advances toward arriving at an early diagnosis to stop the disease process is most important. Understanding new theories of its epidemiology is practice changing. Avoidance of the deformity that predisposes to skin breakdown, prolonged immobility, and more devastating consequences is the ultimate goal and a possibility while using advanced surgical techniques with external fixation and stronger constructs. Medical advances have shown hope of offering other nonsurgical approaches as well, which would make exceedingly prolonged offloading perhaps not the mainstay of treatment in the future.

The treatment of deformities associated with Charcot neuroarthropathy is evolving from a passive approach to one that recognizes the urgency of early recognition.

Avoidance of the cascading events, understanding the etiology, and seeking to reclaim a functional foot should be the primary goals of the treating clinician. Understanding the pathogenesis is complex and the treatment is among the most difficult in foot surgery because the intraoperative, perioperative, and postsurgical treatment is demanding, time consuming, and fraught with challenges in the sick patient who is at increased risk of amputation and premature mortality.

REFERENCES

1. Schade VL, Anderson CA. A literature-based guide to the conservative and surgical management of the acute Charcot foot and ankle. Diabet Foot Ankle 2015; 19(6):26627.
2. Christensen TM, Gade-Rasmussen B, Pedersen LW, et al. Duration of offloading and recurrence rate in Charcot osteoarthropathy treated with less restrictive regimen with removable walker. J Diabetes Complications 2012;26: 430–4.
3. Sinacore DR. Acute Charcot arthropathy in patients with diabetes mellitus: healing times by foot location. J Diabetes Complications 1998;12:287–93.
4. Saltzman CL, Hagy ML, Zimmerman B, et al. How effective is intensive nonoperative initial treatment of patients with diabetes and Charcot arthropathy of the feet? Clin Orthop 2005;435:185–90.
5. Game FL, Catlow R, Jones GR, et al. Audit of acute Charcot's disease in the UK: the CDUK study. Diabetologia 2012;55:32–5.
6. Chantelau E, Richter A, Ghassem-Zadeh N, et al. "Silent" bone stress injuries in the feet of diabetic patients with polyneuropathy: a report on 12 cases. Arch Orthop Trauma Surg 2007;127:171–7.
7. Bariteau JT, Tenenbaum S, Rabinovich A, et al. Charcot arthropathy of the foot and ankle in patients with idiopathic neuropathy. Foot Ankle Int 2014;35: 996–1001.
8. Fabrin J, Larsen K, Holstein PE. Long-term follow up in diabetic Charcot feet with spontaneous onset. Diabetes Care 2000;23:796–800.
9. Pinzur MS, Evans A. Health-related quality of life in patients with charcot foot. Am J Orthop 2003;32(10):492–6.
10. Van Baal J, Hubbard R, Game F, et al. Mortality associated with acute Charcot foot and neuropathic foot ulceration. Diabetes Care 2010;33:1086–9.
11. Suder NC, Wukich DK. Prevalence of diabetic neuropathy in patients undergoing foot and ankle surgery. Foot Ankle Spec 2012;5:97–100.
12. Anthony ML, Cravey KS, Atway SA. Development of Charcot neuroarthropathy in diabetic patients who received kidney or kidney-pancreas transplants. J Foot Ankle Surg 2019;58(3):475–9.
13. Yu TM, Lin CL, Chang SN, et al. Osteoporosis and fractures after solid organ transplantation: a nationwide population-based cohort study. Mayo Clin Proc 2014;89(7):888–95.
14. Dounousi E, Leivaditis K, Eleftheriadis T, et al. Osteoporosis after renal transplantation. Int Urol Nephrol 2015;47(3):503–11.
15. Jansen RB, Svendsen OL. A review of bone metabolism and developments in medical treatment of the diabetic Charcot foot. J Diabetes Complications 2018;32:708–12.
16. Pasquier J, Spurgeon M, Badic M, et al. Whole-methylome analysis of circulating monocytes in acute diabetic Charcot foot reveals differentially methylated genes involved in the formation of osteoclasts. Epigenomics 2019;11(3):281–96.

17. Chen P, Miller PD, Rocker R, et al. Increase in BMC correlate with improvements in bone microarchitecture with teriparatide treatment in post-menopausal women with osteoporosis. J Bone Miner Res 2007;22:1173–80.
18. Mabilleau G, Edmonds ME. Role of neuropathy on fracture healing in Charcot neuro-osteoarthropathy. J Musculoskelet Neuronal Interact 2010;10:84–91.
19. Rastogi A, Hajela A, Prakash M, et al. Teriparatide (recombinant human parathyroid hormone 1-34 increases foot bone remodeling in diabetic chronic Charcot neuroarthropathy: a randomized double-blind placebo-controlled study. J Diabetes 2019. https://doi.org/10.1111/1753-0407.12902.
20. Jeffcoate WJ, Game F, Cavanagh PR. The role of proinflammatory cytokines in the cause of neuropathic osteoarthropathy (acute Charcot foot) in diabetes. Lancet 2005;366:2058–61.
21. Blume PA, Sumpio B, Schmidt B, et al. Charcot neuroarthropathy of the foot and ankle diagnosis and management strategies. In: Blume PA, Zgonis T, editors. Clinics in podiatric medicine and surgery, vol. 31 2014;. p. 1, 51-72.
22. Christensen TM, Simonsen L, Holstein PE, et al. Sympathetic neuropathy in diabetes mellitus patients does not elicit Charcot osteoarthropathy. J Diabetes Complications 2011;25:320–4.
23. Papanas N, Maltezos E. Etiology, pathophysiology and classifications of the diabetic Charcot foot. Diabet Foot ankle 2013;4:208–72.
24. Edmonds ME, Clarke MB, Newton S, et al. Increased uptake of bone radiopharmaceutical in diabetic neuropathy. Q J Med 1985;57:843–55.
25. Barwick AL, de Jonge XA, Tessier JW, et al. The effect of diabetic neuropathy o foot bones: a systematic review and meta-analysis. Diabet Med 2014;31:136–47.
26. Petrova NL, Foster AVM, Edmonds ME. Calcaneal bone mineral density in patients with Charcot neuropathic osteoarthropathy; differences between type 1 and type 2 diabetes. Diabet Med 2005;22:756–61.
27. Sinacore DR, Hastings MK, Bohnert KL, et al. Inflammatory osteolysis in diabetic neuropathic (Charcot) arthropathies of the foot. Phys Ther 2008;88:1399–407.
28. Jirkovská A, Kasalicky P, Boucek P, et al. Calcaneal ultrasonometry in patients with Charcot osteoarthropathy and its relationship with densitometry in the lumbar spine and femoral neck and with markers of bone turnover. Diabet Med 2001;18:495–500.
29. Clasen S. Is diabetic Charcot foot related to lower limb osteopaenia? Foot Ankle Surg 2000;6(4):255–9.
30. Sinacore DR, Bohnert KL, Hastings MK, et al. Persistent inflammation with pedal osteolysis 1 year after Charcot neuropathic osteoarthropathy. J Diabetes Complications 2017;31:1014–20.
31. Witzke KA, Vinik AI, Grant LM, et al. Loss of RAGE defense: a cause of Charcot neuroarthropathy? Diabetes Care 2011;34:1617–21.
32. Jansen RB, Christensen TM, Bűlow J, et al. Bone mineral density and markers of bone turnover and inflammation in diabetes patients with or without a Charcot foot: an 8.5 year prospective case-control study. J Diabetes Complications 2018;32(2):164–70.
33. Christensen TM, Bűlow J, Simonsen L, et al. Bone mineral density in diabetes mellitus patients with and without a Charcot foot. Clin Physiol Funct Imaging 2010;30:130–4.
34. Vestergaard P. Discrepancies in bone mineral density and fracture risk in patients with type 1 and type 2 diabetes—a meta-analysis. Osteoporos Int 2007;18:427–44.

35. DeShields SC, Cunningham TD. Comparison of osteoporosis in US adults with type 1 and type 2 diabetes mellitus. J Endocrinol Invest 2018;41(9):1051–60.
36. Saller A, Maggi S, Romanato G, et al. Diabetes and osteoporosis. Aging Clin Exp Res 2008;20:280–9.
37. Ma L, Oei L, Jiang L, et al. Association between bone mineral density and type 2 diabetes mellitus: a meta-analysis of observational studies. Eur J Epidemiol 2012;27:319.
38. Sundararaghavan V, Mazur MM, Evans B, et al. Diabetes and bone health: latest evidence and clinical implications. Ther Adv Musculoskelet Dis 2017;9:67–74.
39. Vestergaard P, Rejnmark L, Mosekilde L. Diabetes and its complications and their relationship with risk of fracture in type 1 and 2 diabetes. Calcif Tissue Int 2009;84:45–55.
40. Napoli N, Strotmeyer ES, Ensrud KE, et al. Fracture risk in diabetic elderly men: the MrOS study. Diabetologia 2014;57:2057–65.
41. Herbst SA, Jones KB, Saltzman CL. Pattern of diabetic neuropathic arthropathy associated with the peripheral bone mineral density. J Bone Joint Surg Br 2004; 86-B:378-83.
42. La Fontaine J, Shibuya N, Sampson HW, et al. Trabecular quality and cellular characteristics of normal, diabetic, and Charcot bone. J Foot Ankle Surg 2011;50:648–53.
43. Jeffcoate WJ. Theories concerning the pathogenesis of the acute Charcot foot suggest future therapy. Curr Diab Rep 2005;5:430–5.
44. Rogers LC, Frykberg RG, Armstrong DG, et al. The Charcot foot in diabetes. J Am Podiatr Med Assoc 2011;101:437–46.
45. Mabilleau G, Petrova NL, Edmonds ME, et al. Increased osteoclastic activity in acute Charcot's osteoarthropathy: the role of receptor activator of nuclear factor-kappaB ligand. Diabetologia 2008;51:1035–40.
46. Pasquier J, Thomas B, Hoarau-Vechot J, et al. Circulating microparticles in acute diabetic Charcot foot exhibit a high content of inflammatory cytokines, and support monocyte-to-osteoclast cell induction. Sci Rep 2017;7(1):16450.
47. Gough Z, Abraha H, Li F, et al. Measurement of markers of osteoclast and osteoblast activity in patients with acute and chronic diabetic Charcot neuroarthropathy. Diabet Med 1997;14(7):527–31.
48. Petrova NL, Dew TK, Musto RL, et al. Inflammatory and bone turnover markers in a cross-sectional and prospective study of acute Charcot osteoarthropathy. Diabet Med 2015;32:267–73.
49. Folestad A, Ålund M, Asteberg S, et al. IL-17 cytokines in bone healing of diabetic Charcot arthropathy patients: a prospective 2 year follow-up study. J Foot Ankle Res 2015;8:39.
50. Folestad A, Ålund M, Asteberg S, et al. Offloading treatment is linked to activation of proinflammatory cytokines and start of bone repair and remodeling in Charcot arthropathy patients. J Foot Ankle Res 2015;8:72.
51. Divyateja H, Shu KSS, Pearson RG, et al. Local and systemic concentration of pro-inflammatory cytokines, osteoprotegerin, sRANKL and bone turnover markers in acute Charcot foot and in controls. Diabetologia 2011;54:S11–2.
52. Baumhauer JF, O'Keefe RJ, Schon LC, et al. Cytokine-induced osteoclastic bone resorption in Charcot arthropathy: an immunohistochemical study. Foot Ankle Int 2006;27:797–800.
53. Uccioli L, Sinistro A, Almeerighi C, et al. Proinflammatory modulation of the surface and cytokine phenotype of monocytes in patients with acute Charcot foot. Diabetes Care 2010;33:350–5.

54. Sattler AM, Schopper M, Schaefer JR, et al. Novel aspects of RANK ligand and osteoprotegerin in osteoporosis and vascular disease. Calcif Tissue Int 2004;74: 103–6.

55. Hofbauer LC, Schoppet M. Clinical implications of the osteoprotegerin/RANKL/ RANK system for bone and vascular diseases. JAMA 2004;292:490–5.

56. Ndip A, Williams A, Jude EB, et al. The RANKL/RANK/OPG signaling pathway mediates medial arterial calcification in diabetic Charcot neuroarthropathy. Diabetes 2011;60:2187–96.

57. Petrova NL, Petrov PK, Edmonds ME, et al. Novel use of a Dektak 150 surface profiler unmasks differences in resorption pit profiles between control and Charcot patient osteoclasts. Calcif Tissue Int 2014;94(4):403–11.

58. Connors JC, Hardy MA, Kishman LL, et al. Charcot pathogenesis: a study of in vivo gene expression. J Foot Ankle Surg 2018;57(6):1067–72.

59. Bergamini A, Bolacchi F, Pesce CD, et al. Expression of the receptor activator of nuclear factor-κβ ligand in peripheral blood mononuclear cells in patients with acute Charcot neuroarthropathy. Int J Med Sci 2016;13:875–80.

60. Johnson-Lynn SE, McCaskie AW, Coll AP, et al. Neuroarthropathy in diabetes: pathogenesis of Charcot arthropathy. Bone Joint Res 2018;7:373–8.

61. Mabilleau G, Petrova N, Edmonds ME, et al. Number of circulating CD14-positive cells and the serum levels of TNF-α are raised in acute Charcot foot. Diabetes Care 2011;34:e33.

62. Udagawa N, Takahashi N, Akatsu T, et al. Origin of osteoclasts: mature monocytes and macrophages are capable of differentiating into osteoclasts under a suitable microenvironment prepared by bone marrow-derived stromal cells. Proc Natl Acad Sci U S A 1990;87(18):7260–4.

63. Rogers MJ. New insights into the molecular mechanisms of action of bisphosphonates. Curr Pharm Des 2003;9:2643–58.

64. Jude EB, Selby PL, Burgess J, et al. Bisphosphonates in the treatment of Charcot neuroarthropathy: a double-blind randomised controlled trial. Diabetologia 2001;44:2032–7.

65. Pitocco D, Ruotolo V, Caputo S, et al. Six-month treatment with alendronate in acute Charcot neuroarthropathy: a randomized controlled trial. Diabetes Care 2005;28:1214–5.

66. Jeffcoate WJ. Charcot foot syndrome. Diabet Med 2015;32:76–7.

67. Richard JL, Almasri M, Schuldiner S. Treatment of active Charcot foot with bisphosphonates: a systematic review of the literature. Diabetologia 2012;55: 1258–64.

68. Wukich DK, Sung W. Charcot arthropathy of the foot and ankle: modern concepts and management review. J Diabetes Complications 2009;23:409–26.

69. Bem R, Jirkovska A, Fejfarova V, et al. Intranasal calcitonin in the treatment of acute Charcot neuroosteoarthropathy: a randomized controlled trial. Diabetes Care 2006;29:1392–4.

70. La Fontaine J, Harkless LB, Sylvia VL, et al. Levels of endothelial nitric oxide synthase and calcitonin gene-related peptide in the Charcot foot: a pilot study. J Foot Ankle Surg 2008;47:424–9.

71. Busch-Westbroek TE, Delpeut K, Balm R, et al. Effect of single dose of RANKL antibody treatment on acute Charcot neuro-osteoarthropathy of the foot. Diabetes Care 2018;41:e21–2.

72. Zampa V, Bargellini I, Rizzo L, et al. Role of dynamic MRI in the follow-up of acute Charcot foot in patients with diabetes mellitus. Skeletal Radiol 2011;40: 991–9.

73. Hőpfner S, Krolak C, Kessler S, et al. Preoperative imaging of Charcot neuro-arthropathy: does the additional application of (18)F-FDG-PET make sense? Nuklearmedizin 2006;45:15–20.

74. Basu S, Chryssikos T, Houseni M, et al. Potential role of FDG PET in the setting of diabetic neuro-osteoarthropathy: can it differentiate uncomplicated Charcot's neuroarthropathy from osteomyelitis and soft-tissue infection? Nucl Med Commun 2007;28:465–72.

75. Ranachowska C, Lass P, Korzon-Burakowska A, et al. Diagnostic imaging of the diabetic foot. Nucl Med Rev Cent East Eur 2010;13:18–22.

76. Madan SS, Pai DR. Charcot neuroarthropathy of the foot and ankle. Orthop Surg 2013;5:86–93.

77. Zhuang H, Duarte PS, Pourdehand M, et al. Exclusion of chronic osteomyelitis with F-18 fluorodeoxyglucose positron emission tomographic imaging. Clin Nucl Med 2000;25:281–4.

78. Foster AV. Problems with the nomenclature of Charcot's osteoarthropathy. Diabet Foot Ankle 2005;8:37–9.

79. Hockenbury RT, Gruttadauria M, McKinney I. Use of implantable bone growth stimulation in Charcot ankle arthrodesis. Foot Ankle Int 2007;28:971–6.

80. Petrisor B, Lau JT. Electrical bone stimulation: an overview and its use in high risk and Charcot foot and ankle reconstructions. Foot Ankle Clin 2005;10:609–20, vii-viii.

81. Saxena A, DiDomenico LA, Widtfeldt A, et al. Implantable electrical bone stimulation for arthrodesis of the foot and ankle in high-risk patients: a multicenter study. J Foot Ankle Surg 2005;44:450–4.

82. Strauss E, Gonya G. Adjunct low intensity ultrasound in Charcot neuroarthropathy. Clin Orthop Relat Res 1998;(349):132–8.

83. Siddiqui NA, LaPorta GA. Midfoot charcot reconstruction. Clin Podiatr Med Surg 2018;35(4):509–20.

84. Burns PR, Wukich DK. Surgical reconstruction of the Charcot rearfoot and ankle. Clin Podiatr Med Surg 2008;25(1):95–120.

85. Stapleton JJ, Zgonis T. Surgical reconstruction of the diabetic Charcot foot: internal, external or combined fixation? Clin Podiatr Med Surg 2012;12:425–33.

86. Ulbrecht JS, Wukich DK. The Charcot foot: medical and surgical therapy. Curr Diab Rep 2008;8(6):444–51.

87. Kroin E, Chaharbakhshi EO, Schiff A, et al. Improvement in quality of life following operative correction of midtarsal charcot foot deformity. Foot Ankle Int 2018;39(7):808–11.

88. Elmarsafi T, Anghel EL, Sinkin J, et al. Risk factors associated with major lower extremity amputation after osseous diabetic Charcot reconstruction. J Foot Ankle Surg 2019;58(2):295–300.

89. Rettedal D, Parker A, Popchak A, et al. Prognostic scoring system for patients undergoing reconstructive foot and ankle surgery for Charcot neuroarthropathy: the charcot reconstruction preoperative prognostic score. J Foot Ankle Surg 2018;57(3):451–5.

90. Eichenholtz SN. Charcot joints. Springfield (MA): Charles C. Thomas; 1966.

91. Shibata T, Tada K, Hashizume C. The results or arthrodesis of the ankle for leprotic neuroarthropathy. J Bone Joint Surg Am 1990;72:749–56.

92. Yu GV, Hudson JR. Evaluation and treatment of Stage 0 Charcot's neuroarthropathy of the foot and ankle. J Am Podiatr Med Assoc 2002;92:210–20.

93. Sella EJ, Barrette CJ. Staging of Charcot neuroarthropathy along the medial column of the foot in the diabetic patient. Foot Ankle Surg 1999;38(1):34–40.

94. Mittlmeier T, Klaue K, Haar P, et al. Should one consider primary surgical reconstruction in Charcot arthropathy of the feet? Clin Orthop Relat Res 2010;468(4): 1002–11.

95. Simon SR, Tejwani SG, Wilson DL, et al. Arthrodesis as an early alternative to nonoperative management of Charcot arthropathy of the diabetic foot. J Bone Joint Surg Am 2000;82-A(7):939–50.

96. Lamm BM, Gottlieb HD, Paley D. A two-stage percutaneous approach to Charcot diabetic foot reconstruction. J Foot Ankle Surg 2010;49(6):517–22.

97. DiDomenico L, Flynn Z, Reed M. Treating Charcot arthropathy is a challenge: explaining why my treatment algorithm has changed. Clin Podiatr Med Surg 2018;35(1):105–21.

98. Greenhagen RM, Johnson AR, Bevilacqua NJ. Gastrocnemius recession or tendo-Achilles lengthening for equinus deformity in the diabetic foot? Clin Podiatr Med Surg 2012;29(3):413–24.

99. Ramanujum CL, Facaros Z, Zgonis T. External fixation for surgical off-loading of diabetic soft tissue reconstruction. Clin Podiatr Med Surg 2011;28(1):211–6.

100. Maluf KS, Mueller MJ, Strube MJ, et al. Tendon Achilles lengthening for the treatment of neuropathic ulcers causes a temporary reduction in forefoot pressure associated with changes in plantar flexor power rather than ankle motion during gait. J Biomech 2004;37:897–906.

101. Sanders LJ, Frykberg RG. The Charcot foot. In: Frykberg RG, editor. The high risk foot in diabetes mellitus. New York: Churchill Livingstone; 1991. p. 325–35.

102. Orendurff MS, Rohr ES, Sangeorzan BJ, et al. An equinus deformity of the ankle accounts for only a small amount of the increased forefoot plantar pressure in patients with diabetes. J Bone Joint Surg Br 2006;88(1):65–8.

103. Laborde JM. Midfoot ulcers treated with tendon lengthenings. Foot Ankle Int 2009;30:842–6.

104. Laborde JM, Philbin TM, Chandler PJ, et al. Preliminary results of primary gastrocnemius-soleus recession for midfoot Charcot arthropathy. Foot Ankle Spec 2015;9(2):140–4.

105. Belczyk R, Ramanujam CL, Capobianco CM, et al. Combined midfoot arthrodesis, muscle flap coverage, and circular external fixation for the chronic ulcerated Charcot deformity. Foot Ankle Spec 2009;3(1):40–4.

106. Ramanujam CL, Zgonis T. Versatility of intrinsic muscle flaps for the diabetic charcot foot. Clin Podiatr Med Surg 2012;29(2):323–6.

107. Catanzariti AR, Mendicino R, Haverstock B. Ostectomy for diabetic neuroarthropathy involving the midfoot. J Foot Ankle Surg 2000;39:291–300.

108. Armstrong DG, Lavery LA. Elevated peak plantar pressures in patients who have Charcot arthropathy. J Bone Joint Surg Am 1998;80:365–9.

109. Brodsky JW, Rouse AM. Exostectomy for symptomatic bony prominences in diabetic Charcot feet. Clin Orthop 1993;296:21–6.

110. Laurinaviciene R, Kirketerp-Moeller K, Holstein PE. Exostectomy for chronic mid-foot plantar ulcer in Charcot deformity. J Wound Care 2008;17:53–9.

111. Brodsky JW. The diabetic foot. In: Coughlin MJ, Mann RA, Saltzman CL, editors. Surgery of the foot and ankle. Philadelphia: Mosby Elsevier; 2007. p. 1281–368.

112. Wukich DK, Raspovic KM, Hobizal KB, et al. Radiographic analysis of diabetic midfoot Charcot neuroarthropathy with and without midfoot ulceration. Foot Ankle Int 2014;35(11):1108–15.

113. Dayton P, Feilmeier M, Thompson M, et al. Comparison of complications for internal and external fixation for Charcot reconstruction: a systematic review. J Foot Ankle Surg 2015;54(6):1072–5.

114. Lowery J, Woods JB, Armstrong DG, et al. Surgical management of charcot neuroarthropathy of the foot and ankle: a systematic review. Foot Ankle Int 2012;33:113–21.
115. Bisaccia M, Vicente CI, Meccariello, et al. The history of external fixation, a revolution idea for the treatment of limb's traumatized and deformities: from Hippocrates to today. Can Open Orthop Traumatol J 2016;3(4):1–9.
116. Watson JT. Principles of external fixation. In: Court-Brown CM, Heckman JD, McQueen MM, et al, editors. Rockwood and Green's fractures in adults. 8th edition. Philadelphia: Lippincott Williams & Wilkins; 2010. p. 206–40.
117. Kowalski M, Schemitsch EH, Harrington RM, et al. Comparative biomechanical evaluation of different external fixation sidebars: stainless-steel tubes versus carbon fiber rods. J Orthop Trauma 1996;10:470–5.
118. Moss DP, Tejwani NC. Biomechanics of external fixation: a review of the literature. Bull NYU Hosp Jt Dis 2007;65(4):294–9.
119. Sammarco JV. Superconstructs in the treatment of charcot foot deformity: plantar plating, locked plating, and axial screw fixation. Foot Ankle Clin 2009; 14(3):393–407.
120. Pope E, Takemoto R, Kummer F, et al. Midfoot fusion: a biomechanical comparison of plantar planting vs intramedullary screws. Foot Ankle Int 2013;34(3):409–13.
121. Grant WP, Garcia-Lavin S, Sabo R. Beaming the columns for Charcot diabetic foot reconstruction: a retrospective analysis. J Foot Ankle Surg 2011;50(2):182–9.
122. Wukich DK, Mallory BR, Suder NC, et al. Tibiotalocalcaneal arthrodesis using retrograde intramedullary nail fixation: comparison of patients with and without diabetes mellitus. J Foot Ankle Surg 2015;54(5):876–82.
123. Noonan T, Pinzur M, Paxinos O, et al. Tibiotalocalcaneal arthrodesis with a retrograde intramedullary nail: a biomechanical analysis of the effect of nail length. Foot Ankle Int 2005;26(4):304–8.
124. Jones CP. Beaming of Charcot foot reconstruction. Foot Ankle Int 2015;36(7):853–9.
125. Brandão RA, Weber JS, Larson D, et al. New fixation methods for the treatment of the diabetic foot: beaming, external fixation, and beyond. Clin Podiatr Med Surg 2018;35(1):63–76.
126. Garchar D, DiDomenico LA, Klaue K. Reconstruction of Lisfranc joint dislocations secondary to Charcot neuroarthropathy using a plantar plate. J Foot Ankle Surg 2013;52(3):295–7.
127. Marks RM, Parks BG, Schon LC. Midfoot fusion technique for neuroarthropathic feet: biomechanical analysis and rationale. Foot Ankle Int 1998;19(8):507–10.
128. Jastifer JR. Topical review: locking plate technology in foot and ankle surgery. Foot Ankle Int 2014;35(5):512–8.
129. Cullen AB, Curtiss S, Lee MA. Biomechanical comparison of polyaxial and uniaxial locking plate fixation in a proximal tibial gap model. J Orthop Trauma 2009; 23(7):507–13.

Diagnosis and Treatment Options for Inflammatory Skin Conditions of the Lower Extremity

Tracey C. Vlahovic, DPM, FFPM, RCPS (Glasg)

KEYWORDS

- Plantar psoriasis • Eczema • Lichen planus • Topical steroid

KEY POINTS

- To provide a systematic approach to examining and treating inflammatory skin conditions.
- To discuss the most common skin conditions seen in the podiatric practitioner's office.
- To discuss the first-line treatment for inflammatory skin disorders.

INTRODUCTION

The lower extremity presents several challenges from a dermatologic standpoint: there are different anatomic areas that not only vary (dorsum foot, plantar foot, anterior tibia, posterior leg, interdigital skin, nail unit) from a stratum corneum thickness and histologic standpoint but are also subject to trauma that is unique (shoe gear, gait cycle). This creates dermatologic presentations that can be frustrating to the practitioner and the patient, as lesions may present differently or even in isolation from other areas of the body. Attention to appropriate diagnosis and management is always warranted but should be especially vigilant to those treating issues of the lower extremity. This article reviews diagnosis and treatment of the most common skin and nail conditions of the foot and ankle.

Observe

On entering the treatment room, the practitioner should notice color, shape, and size in addition to laterality of the lesions on the lower extremity. Primary and secondary lesions (**Box 1**) should be used to describe the rash appropriately both in the chart and in correspondence to other physicians. When looking at the shape of the lesions,

The author has nothing to disclose.
Department of Podiatric Medicine, Temple University School of Podiatric Medicine, 148 North 8th Street, Philadelphia, PA 19107, USA
E-mail address: traceyv@temple.edu
; @drchacha (T.C.V.)

podiatric.theclinics.com

Box 1
Primary and secondary skin lesions

Primary Skin Lesions:
  Macule
  Patch
  Plaque
  Nodule
  Vesicle
  Bullae
  Wheal
  Telangiectasia

Secondary Skin Lesions:
  Ulcer
  Atrophy
  Scale
  Crust
  Erosion
  Excoriation
  Scar
  Lichenification

---

it is helpful to determine if they were self-induced by the patient (excoriation by a fingernail) or are a manifestation of a systemic issue (psoriasis). One should document if the lesions are plantar foot, dorsal foot, or headed proximally on the lower leg. Nail involvement should be noted and examined with the patient's knees bent with feet flat on the examining surface. Finally, the fingernails and dorsum and palmar aspects of the hands should be examined as many skin dermatoses and nail dystrophies mirror the pedal involvement there.

Ask

Questions that will help form differential diagnoses should be asked while completing the physical examination of the skin. Often, the patient will answer a question that will help direct the diagnosis. Beyond asking the history of present illness, past medical history, and family history, the podiatric physician should consider asking if there is a personal or family history of allergic rhinitis, sensitive skin, asthma, joint pain, or skin cancer. The patient should be asked if he has ever seen a dermatologist before and if he has any skin lesions or "rashes" anywhere else on the body that may or may not be like what is seen on the feet. Unfortunately, most patients do not correlate what is happening on the rest of the body to what is manifesting on the plantar aspect of the feet or nails. It is the physician's responsibility to ask the questions in order to make that connection. It is helpful to ask if the skin has ever been biopsied (eg, "did you have a piece of skin removed that was sent to a laboratory?"). A skin scraping for KOH that was completed by another physician does not count as a proper biopsy to base the diagnosis on, as a biopsy of inflammatory skin disorders should include the epidermis, dermis, and some subcutaneous tissue from a histopathology perspective. Other questions to consider would be asking patients the color of socks they wear (azo dyes in blue socks can be a potential allergen), occupation, and any associated daily hazards. Also, the practitioner may inquire about both over-the-counter folk remedy and homeopathic or natural treatment options they have tried. In order to plan for a possible in-office biopsy visit, it is important to determine the natural progression of the lesions in question and the location of the newest crop of lesions.

Now that basic observation and questioning have occurred, it is important to delve into the chief complaint and examine the skin fully. Common skin signs of inflammation are calor (heat), rubor (redness), tumor (swelling), and pruritis (itching) that ultimately point to skin barrier dysfunction. The skin barrier, which is stratum corneum with the lipid-enriched extracellular matrix surrounding the corneocytes, is the body's protective wall, and it regulates homeostasis and transepidermal water loss and prevents entry of foreign particles and pathogens into the body. Transepidermal water loss is the newest target in the dermatologic pharmaceutical armamentarium in order to reduce skin flares.

Apply an Algorithm

To begin formulating a differential diagnosis, the physician may consider a basic algorithm to follow for treating the most common skin disorders encountered in the office: is it a plaque, scale, or zebra? (**Box 2**) A well-defined and geometric-shaped plaque is often psoriasis, but eczema and lichen planus also must be considered. Circular, serpiginous scales are most often tinea, but xerosis should be ruled out. Remember that tinea pedis is KOH positive and may involve both the interspaces and the plantar foot. Any papules, vesicles, or other skin markings are considered "zebras" for this algorithm's purpose.

Following an algorithm, the most common inflammatory skin conditions the podiatric practitioner will encounter are as follows:

Plaque

Plantar psoriasis may appear alone, in combination with palmar involvement, or in combination with psoriatic lesions elsewhere on the body. Psoriasis can develop either in childhood or as an adult. Plaque psoriasis, the most common type, presents as an erythematous plaque with a silvery scale. These lesions are geographic, bilateral, and symmetric, which typically occur on the extensor surfaces. The plaques can also be pruritic and affect joints as well as the nails during the progression of the disease. Besides plaque psoriasis, pustular psoriasis appears as sterile pustules on the plantar foot. Plantar plaque and pustular psoriasis are frequently misdiagnosed as either vesicular or moccasin tinea pedis. Because of the fissuring that often accompanies psoriatic plaques, it has also been misdiagnosed as xerosis. If the patient's current treatment consists of either an oral or a topical antifungal and the skin condition is not improved within the appropriate time frame, a biopsy of the skin in order to determine if a topical steroid should be prescribed is warranted. Also, if the patient only presents with an onychomycosis-like nail involvement and has failed oral antifungals, a diagnosis of psoriatic nail disease should be considered. Another clue to aid in the diagnosis of psoriatic nails includes examining for the presence of erythema periungual, onycholysis, and pitting.[1] Patients may also present with the arthritic

---

Box 2
Algorithm

Plaque: consider psoriasis, lichen planus, eczema

Scale: consider xerosis, tinea pedis, ichthyosis, noninflamed to mildly inflamed psoriasis and eczema

Zebra blisters: bullous diabeticorum, pemphigus, drug reaction
   Target lesions: erythema multiforme minor, drug reaction

component of psoriasis, which may manifest in dactylitis of the digits (sausage toes), enthesitis of the Achilles tendon, and distal interphalangeal joint involvement.

Case example

A 23-year-old male patient presents with a pruritic and scaly plantar rash (**Figs. 1** and **2**) that was misdiagnosed as tinea pedis at the Emergency Department (ED). He presented with painful fissures on his feet that prevented him from walking properly. He was given oral ketoconazole at the ED and then referred to the office. A punch biopsy was taken confirming the clinical suspicion of psoriasis, and topical corticosteroid therapy was implemented. The patient healed uneventfully from the acute flare and presents periodically for maintenance treatment (end of case).

If a patient presents with circular papules or plaques with little or no scale that extend proximally from the foot, a differential diagnosis of psoriasis is lichen planus. Lichen planus is characteristic of the "P's": plentiful, pruritic, purple, polished, popular, and planar lesions that are bilateral and symmetric. Wickham's striae, the fine white

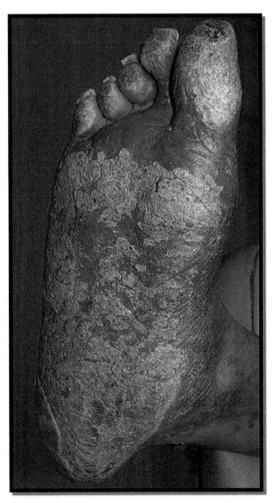

Fig. 1. Psoriasis on first presentation.

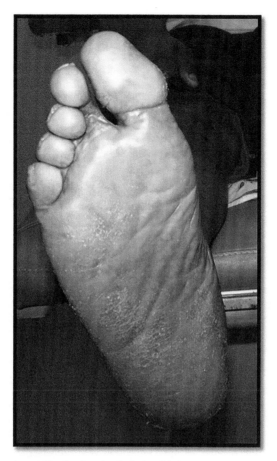

Fig. 2. Psoriasis on 1 month of using topical steroid therapy.

lacy overlay on the plaques, may also be seen. This skin condition can be so pruritic that activities of daily living may be compromised. It may also affect the toenails, appearing anywhere from a proximal subungual onychomycosis-like presentation to a thinning of the nail with a "wing" of skin or pterygium pointing distally (**Fig. 3**).[1] Nail involvement should be treated immediately, as it can irreversibly scar the nail unit. Lichen planus can also form lesions in the mouth.[2]

Case example
A young man presented with numerous small plaques and papules that were extremely pruritic (**Fig. 4**). He had been diagnosed with tinea pedis and had tried over-the-counter antifungals with no improvement. During his office visit, the extent of involvement of the nails and oral cavity were noted, and a diagnosis of lichen planus was made (end of case).

In addition to psoriasis and lichen planus, a scaly erythematous rash with fissures could also be an eczematous reaction pattern. Defined plaques may or may not be present, but eczema should be a differential diagnosis when considering psoriasis. An eczematous reaction that is often seen is atopic dermatitis. This is usually inherited, as patients will present with a personal or family history of asthma, hay fever, and skin

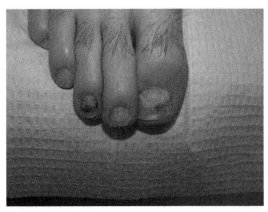

Fig. 3. Nail involvement in lichen planus.

rash appropriate for their age. It is often described as an "itch that gets a rash" and cannot be described as having a primary lesion as is the case with psoriasis.[3] Atopic dermatitis, as the other forms of eczema, can be described as having an acute, sub-acute, and chronic stage of the disease. During the acute phase, patients experience intense pruritus with an erythematous scaling and oozing skin rash. Clinically, this can also appear as dry skin eczema, contact dermatitis, stasis dermatitis, or even a dermatophyte infection.

Subacute forms of atopic dermatitis present with less pruritus, erythema, scaling, and fissured skin rash. Chronic eczema presents with pruritus, hyper- and hypopig-mented plaques of previous inflamed skin, and scaly and lichenified skin. Because of the severe skin barrier disruption in all forms of atopic dermatitis, these patients are susceptible to secondary bacterial infections, and this should be considered in the treatment plan. Overall, differential diagnosis for atopic dermatitis includes tinea pedis, contact dermatitis, lichen simplex chronicus (a chronic form of atopic), and dys-hidrosiform eczema.[3]

If the patient does not have the "triad" of atopic dermatitis, other types of eczema should be considered. Allergic contact dermatitis can occur when a patient has devel-oped sensitivity to a product (detergent, soap, glue, dye) after using it for a length of

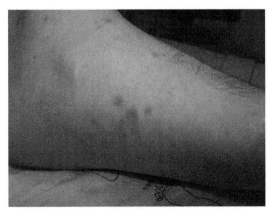

Fig. 4. Pedal lichen planus.

time. Allergic contact dermatitis is a result of an antigen-antibody reaction that presents 8 to 28 days after initial introduction to the allergen. Contrary to belief, a contact dermatitis can occur on the plantar feet and does not have to be bilateral and symmetric. The patch test done in an allergist or dermatologist's office will assist in pinpointing the allergen causing the reaction. When patients have a history of chronic venous insufficiency with skin that becomes indurated, inflamed, and pruritic, venous stasis dermatitis is the standard diagnosis. Because stasis dermatitis is the most common cause of an id reaction on the palmar aspect of the hand, it is important for the physician to examine the hands to aid in the diagnosis. Lastly, dyshidrotic eczema is a specific condition that should not be an overall term applied to any inflamed skin condition. Contrary to its name, it is not linked to sweat gland dysfunction.[4] Dyshidrotic eczema characteristically has pruritic tapioca pudding-like blisters on the palmar aspect of the hands with minimal foot involvement.[4] This can be a self-limiting condition; however, most patients have debilitating pain and fissuring that can be difficult to treat.

Case example
A female patient presented with denuded and inflamed skin on the anterior tibia (**Fig. 5**). She reported this began after the use of triple antibiotic ointment. On further history and examination of the patient, a working diagnosis of allergic contact dermatitis to the preservatives in triple antibiotic ointment was made. The drug was removed from the patient's regimen, and topical steroids were given. The patient's inflamed skin resolved in 4 weeks (end of case).

Scale
Xerotic, or dry skin, should have scales present within the skin lines on the plantar foot. Moccasin tinea pedis, on the other hand, usually presents with small serpiginous scales plantar and in the interspaces. The most common form of dry skin that is KOH negative encountered on the lower extremity is termed asteatotic or xerotic eczema. It can also be termed erythema craquele. This is commonly known as "winter itch" due to its increased severity especially during the winter months in the northern part of the United States. Asteatotic eczema commonly presents on the anterior aspect of the leg as pruritic, annular, scaling patches. This condition is frequently misdiagnosed as tinea corporis but will be KOH negative. Asteatotic eczema is also seen in patients with dementia who bathe frequently. Patients can also develop dry,

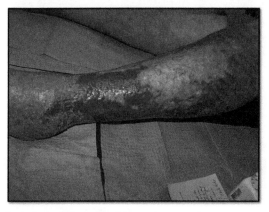

Fig. 5. Allergic contact dermatitis on the leg.

cracked heels plantar, which is known as keratoderma climacterum. In addition to these environmental causes of dry skin, the most common inherited form is ichthyosis vulgaris. These patients present with fish scale–like dryness that may improve with age. Ichthyosis vulgaris can also be acquired and may be associated with diabetes, renal disease, and various types of cancer. Circular scales with serpiginous borders are often diagnosed as tinea pedis, but other skin conditions that present as small circular, scaly rimmed lesions are pityriasis rosea and secondary syphilis. There have also been instances of plantar psoriasis presenting as scaly skin with no erythema.

Case example

A female patient presented to the clinic for a second opinion. She had been previously diagnosed as having xerosis but continued to have extreme pruritus that was not controlled by any topical medication. Her plantar feet had a localized plaque with scale in the medial arch with no underlying erythema (**Fig. 6**). A biopsy helped to diagnose her with psoriasis and the appropriate therapy commenced (end of case).

Zebra

If vesicles, bullae, or other skin lesions are present, the podiatric physician should consider other differential diagnoses. If a diabetic patient presents with tense blisters that seem to appear overnight, it is most likely bullosis diabeticorum.[5] Bullosis diabeticorum may have little inflammation present and may heal uneventfully if the patient does not deroof or scratch them. Bullous pemphigoid, commonly seen in older adults in assisted care facilities, will present with subepidermal blisters that originally were urticarial plaques that turned into tense bullae. These lesions are located widespread throughout the body on flexural surfaces. Nikolsky sign, or exfoliation of the upper layers of epidermis on rubbing of the skin, is negative and these lesions can crust, pigment, but not scar unless excoriated into an ulcer. Pemphigus vulgaris is a chronic disease affecting adults, which can be life threatening due to its lesions beginning in the mouth and affecting the oropharyngeal area. Flaccid bullae then progress to the face, neck, chest, groin, and intertriginous areas. These are tender lesions and are usually Nikolsky sign positive.

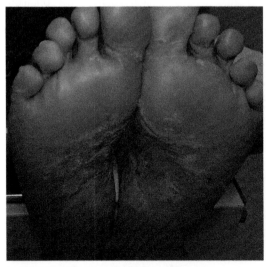

Fig. 6. Psoriatic scale plantar without underlying erythema.

If patients have target lesions with 3 zones of color (center lesion surrounded by a clear zone and followed by a red border) associated with circular papules and/or plaques with mild scaling, one must consider erythema multiforme minor. This is associated after a manifestation of herpes simplex (recent cold sore or genital lesion) and the target lesions may present on the feet.[6] Drug reactions may also present as targetlike lesions with less defined target zones of color on the lower extremity.

FIRST-LINE TREATMENT OPTIONS

When treating a condition that is fungal, bacterial, or inflammatory in nature, the podiatric practitioner should use the appropriate drug, but if one is unsure of the cause, a biopsy (punch or incisional) of the skin lesion should be performed. Inflammatory skin conditions often warrant a topical corticosteroid therapy as a first-line method in treatment. It is useful to avoid combination steroid-antifungal drugs or methylprednisolone dose packs as these may create a quick fix but ultimately can cause frustration for the patient. The rebound effect from the dose pack can be potentially debilitating by causing a dermatitis that is worse than the original reaction, and the dose pack itself is not the same as prescribing a true prednisone taper. When in doubt, the first-line therapy for an inflammatory skin dermatosis should be a topical steroid appropriate for the level of inflammation and pruritus present and a skin moisturizer or keratolytic topical (such as urea, lactic acid, or salicylic acid-based preparations).

The stage (acute, subacute, and chronic) of the skin disorder and the length of time the condition present will aid in determining the level of topical steroid needed.

For the severe, acute inflammatory skin concerns, Class I topical corticosteroids should be used for 2 weeks consecutively. Examples of Class I steroids include clobetasol, betamethasone, diflorasone, halobetasol, and fluocinonide. Side effects include skin thinning or atrophy, which can lead to stretch marks, telangiectasias, and hypopigmentation to name a few. It is helpful to titrate down from a Class I steroid to a midpotency preparation after that initial 2-week period. For example, the patient may use a Class I steroid on Monday, Wednesday, and Friday, with the midpotency topical steroid for the days in between. In addition to the topical corticosteroid, a moisturizer that is fragrance free and contains ingredients such as hyaluronic acid, ceramides, or physiologic lipids should be added to decrease transepidermal water loss and decrease flares.[7] If the patient is in the subacute or chronic stage and a topical steroid is warranted for the level of irritation and pruritus present, the practitioner should prescribe the appropriate steroid Class (**Box 3**). The goal in treating inflammatory

---

Box 3
Topical steroid classes

Class I: Ultra-potent

Class II: Potent

Class III: Upper mid-strength

Class IV: Mid-strength

Class V: Lower mid-strength

Class VI: Mild

Class VII: Least potent (over-the-counter hydrocortisone)

Data from National Psoriasis Foundation. Topical Steroids Potency Chart. Available at: https://www.psoriasis.org/about-psoriasis/treatments/topicals/steroids/potency-chart.

conditions is to ultimately have the patient use little to no topical steroid and use the previously mentioned skin moisturizers as maintenance if possible. If the patient does not respond to the topical steroid as predicted, further consideration of other diagnoses should be given, and a biopsy should be planned. If this is not within the comfort zone of the practitioner, he should then refer the patient for a dermatology consult.

Overall, inflammatory skin dermatoses can be challenging and frustrating for both the practitioner and patient. By doing a thorough history and skin examination, the astute practitioner can create a working list of differential diagnoses that can be further changed by both reaction to treatment and of course, a biopsy result. In addition, understanding that lesions on the lower extremity may appear alone or in concert to lesions elsewhere on the body and are subject to mechanical stress and trauma from the gait cycle and shoes is an important consideration to successful diagnosis and management of inflammatory skin lesions on the lower extremity.

REFERENCES

1. Zaiac MN, Daniel CR. Nails in systemic disease. Dermatol Ther 2002;15:99–106.
2. Bolognia JL, Jorizzo JL, Rapini RP. 1st edition. Dermatology, Vol. 1 and 2, 2003.
3. Brenninkmeijer EE, Schram ME, Leeflang MM, et al. Diagnostic criteria for atopic dermatitis: a systematic review. Br J Dermatol 2008;158(4):754–65.
4. Lofgren SM, Warshaw EM. Dyshidrosis: epidemiology, clinical characteristics, and therapy. Dermatitis 2006;17(4):165–81.
5. Cantwell AR Jr, Martz W. Idiopathic bullae in diabetics. Bullosis diabeticorum. Arch Dermatol 1967;96(1):42–4.
6. Huff JC. Erythema multiforme and latent herpes simplex infection. Semin Dermatol 1992;11(3):207–10.
7. Cork MJ, Danby S. Skin barrier breakdown: a renaissance in emollient therapy. Br J Nurs 2009;18(14):872, 874, 876-877.

Opioid Crisis and Acute Pain Management After Foot and Ankle Surgery

Melinda A. Bowlby, DPM, AACFAS[a,b,c,*], Mary E. Crawford, DPM[b,c]

KEYWORDS

• Opioids • Foot • Ankle • Surgery • Pain • Multimodal

KEY POINTS

- Pain became the fifth vital sign in the early 2000s, which in turn led to a considerable increase in the prescription of opioids and contributed to the current opioid crisis.
- Big Pharma—Purdue Pharma—makers of oxycontin, in the mid-1990s, heavily promoted the use of long-acting opioids as a safe and effective pain management strategy with diminished risk of addiction. This led physicians to prescribe these medications with increased frequency.
- Patients are often overprescribed opioid pain medication following foot and ankle surgery, which is considered to be one of the most painful types of surgery. Physicians' pressure to prescribe pain medication is multifactorial.
- There are current national guidelines for chronic opioid prescribing, but guidelines for prescribing opioids for acute pain have not yet been established.
- The use of multimodal pain control can greatly improve overall pain control and decrease opioid consumption. Multimodal pain control may include: regional anesthesia, liposomal bupivacaine, nonsteroidal anti-inflammatory drugs (NSAIDS), acetaminophen, gabapentin, and pregabalin, and/or antihistamines.

HISTORY OF OPIOIDS AND THE OPIOID EPIDEMIC

The history of opioids dates back to many early civilizations who cultivated the opium poppy plant for medicinal and recreational purposes.[1] The opioid epidemic is not new to the United States, and actually began more than 150 years ago.[2] Morphine became widely used in the United States during the Civil War era, after which many soldiers became addicted.[3] Heroin was synthesized from morphine, and sold in

Disclosure: The authors have nothing to disclose.
[a] Department of Orthopedics, Division of Podiatry, Swedish Medical Center, Seattle, WA, USA;
[b] Department of Orthopedics, Division of Podiatry, Providence Medical Center, Everett, WA, USA; [c] Private Practice, The Ankle and Foot Clinic of Everett, 3131 Nassau Street Suite 101, Everett, WA 98201, USA
* Corresponding author. The Ankle and Foot Clinic of Everett, 3131 Nassau Street Suite 101, Everett, WA 98201.
E-mail address: Melinda.bowlby@gmail.com

over-the-counter cough syrups until the Heroin Act in 1924 ended this because of the severe heroin addiction epidemic.[2] Oxycodone became available in 1950 after being approved by the Food and Drug Administration, and since then numerous other opioids have been created with intravenous, oral, and transdermal routes.[1] In 1970, the federal government passed the Controlled Substances Act, and drugs were placed into categories I-V with an attempt to regulate and control the distribution of these drugs (**Table 1**).[4]

Resurgence of the opioid epidemic began when the Veterans Administration and the Joint Commission made pain the fifth vital sign in the early 2000s, which in turn led to a considerable increase in the prescription of opioids.[3,5,6] Pain, at any level, was determined to be unacceptable by patients and the medical community.[5] Patient satisfaction surveys were heavily used and publicized directly linking increased pain to lower patient satisfaction and therefore reduced financial reimbursement to medical institutions and, in turn, to various departments and/or physicians within the hospital system.[3]

Pharmaceutical companies also share the blame for the opioid crisis. Extended-release oxycodone was heavily marketed by Purdue Pharma from the mid-1990s to the early 2000s.[7] Purdue misrepresented the highly addictive potential of the drug, later paying millions of dollars in fines.[7] Opioid prescriptions increased from 164 to 234 million from 2000 to 2010.[5] In the United States alone, the sale of hydrocodone increased by 244% and oxycodone increased by 732% from 1997 to 2006.[8] It is currently estimated that over 2 million Americans are opioid dependent.[9] Sadly, there have been nearly 218,000 American deaths related to opioid abuse from 1999 to 2017.[10]

The opioid epidemic is not unique, but it is most prevalent in the United States because this country consumes approximately 80% of the world's opioid supply.[8,11] In many European countries, patients are infrequently prescribed opioids, and yet report satisfaction with postoperative pain control.[12] When comparing the United States with the Netherlands, 85% of American patients were prescribed opioids compared with 58% of Dutch patients after open reduction and internal fixation of ankle or hip fractures.[13] In the same study, 77% of American patients were discharged with a prescription for opioids, whereas none of the Dutch patients were prescribed narcotics at the time of discharge.[13] It is quite evident that what is considered an acceptable level of pain control sets the culture for patient expectations and opioid prescription use.[13]

Table 1 Scheduled drugs		
Drug schedule	**Potential for abuse**	**Example**
Schedule I	Prohibited illicit drugs	Heroin
Schedule II	High	Morphine Hydromorphone Oxycodone Hydrocodone
Schedule III	Moderate to low	Acetaminophen with codeine
Schedule IV	Low	Tramadol
Schedule V	Very low	Pregabalin

Data from Courtright D. The controlled substances act: how a "big tent" reform became a punitive drug law. Drug and Alcohol Dependence 2004;76:9-15.

OVERPRESCRIBING

Patients have reported that orthopedic surgery, especially foot and ankle surgery, is one of the most painful types of surgery.[14] As such, orthopedic surgeons are one of the highest prescribers of opioids, ranking third of all specialties.[15] Although the amount of opioids consumed after foot and ankle surgery differs by procedure and by patient, there are some patterns that are noteworthy.[15] Younger patients and those having osseous procedures typically require more pain medication than older patients or those undergoing soft tissue procedures only.[15] Patients who are experiencing higher levels of pain preoperatively are also likely to have greater than expected postoperative pain.[14] Also, patients who suffer from depression and anxiety tend to experience more postoperative pain and consume more opioids.[16,17] Likewise, patients who are taking opioids before surgery are at risk for requiring more opioids than expected, and for an extended period, postoperatively.[12]

Because physicians are unsure how much pain medication a patient will require, opioids are often overprescribed. Saini and colleagues[15] found that patients undergoing foot and ankle surgery only used around half of the opioids that were prescribed, consuming a median of 20 pills. Gupta and colleagues[18] found similar results with patients taking, on average, 22.5 pills, and recommended prescribing only 30 pills for patients undergoing foot and ankle surgery. Reducing the amount of opioids prescribed will limit residual medication, which can end up being misused by patients or their friends and family members. In addition, patients should be educated on proper disposal of narcotic medications, because 55.7% of people over the age of 12 years who used opioids recreationally reported that they obtained them initially from family or friends.[8]

PHYSICIANS' PRESSURE TO PRESCRIBE

Postoperative pain control directly correlates to patient satisfaction, which can weigh heavily on physicians' perceived performance and may result in overprescribing of opioids.[19,20] Physicians have admitted to the fear of losing their jobs and often feel conflicted between providing high-quality care and achieving high patient satisfaction scores.[20] Even physicians in private practice may be impacted by patient satisfaction with regard to referrals or online reviews. Physicians may also fear the threat of a lawsuit because of under-prescribing pain medication to a patient postoperatively. Startlingly, there is even a report of a physical medicine and rehabilitation specialist who was shot and killed in his office parking lot by a patient's husband after refusing to prescribe opioids.[21] Although most physicians need not fear for their lives, most physicians do experience pressure to prescribe opioids on a regular basis for a multitude of reasons.

GUIDELINES

The Centers for Disease Control and Prevention (CDC) has issued the most recent guidelines in 2016 for prescribing opioids for chronic pain, defined as pain lasting longer than 3 months.[22] Currently, there is no definition of acute pain or guidelines for managing acute postoperative pain on a national level. Some tenants of the chronic pain guidelines, however, can be applied to acute pain. First and foremost, the benefit of prescribing opioids should outweigh the risk, and, when possible, nonopioid medications should be used initially.[22] It is also important to educate patients on the expectations of pain control and that the goal of postoperative pain control is to prevent excessive pain but is unlikely to achieve a zero pain level on the pain scale.[22]

Risks of pain medications should be discussed with patients, and long-acting extended-release opioids should not be prescribed.[22] Physicians should avoid prescribing opioids in combination with benzodiazepines and educate patients about the increased risk of respiratory depression and death when these 2 medications are combined.[22] Clinicians should prescribe the lowest effective dose and should avoid prescribing more than 90 morphine milligram equivalents (MME) per day.[22] For example, 2 tablets of oxycodone 5 mg, taken every 4 hours, would be 60 mg of oxycodone consumed over 24 hours. Multiply this cumulative dose by the conversion factor of 1.5 and it is equivalent to 90 MME (**Table 2**).[22] Physicians should abide by these guidelines, when feasible, and also review state prescription monitoring programs to verify that patients are not receiving opioids from more than one source.[22] Through these monitoring programs, surgeons can also verify that patients are not misusing their credentials and obtaining opioids through false pretenses or identities.

Physicians rely on evidence-based medicine to establish protocols used in their daily practice, therefore difficulties arise because there are so many gray areas in terms of prescribing opioids for acute pain. Many states are creating opioid guidelines to fill in the blanks in the CDC guidelines. For example, the Washington State Department of Health established opioid prescribing requirements in 2018.[23] Acute pain is defined as 0 to 6 weeks of pain, and subacute pain is defined as 6 to 12 weeks of pain.[23] Patients are limited to a 7-day supply of opioids during the acute pain period.[23] Podiatric physicians are required to obtain a pain management consultation if more than a 120-morphine equivalent dose is being prescribed per day.[23] It is also mandated that prescription monitoring programs are checked for any patient obtaining an opioid prescription.[23] Podiatric physicians are required to provide patient education on the risks, safe storage, and proper disposal of opioids.[23] Many states are also implementing similar guidelines along with prescription take-back programs so that patients can surrender unused pills.

Implementing an opioid contract with patients is one way to educate them about the risks of opioids, as well as to explain the rules of use, such as not combining opioids with alcohol, not sharing opioids, and not obtaining opioids from multiple providers. The American Academy of Orthopedic Surgeons (AAOS) recommends setting a practice policy for the amount of opioids prescribed and their duration of use.[11] AAOS also recommends writing 2 prescriptions with specified refill dates of smaller quantities of opioids for patients who live long distances from the surgeons' office.[11] In the authors' practice, they do not provide patients with postoperative opioid refills for longer than 30 days. If patients require opioid pain medication for longer than 1 month postoperatively, a referral to pain management should be considered.

Table 2
Morphine milligram equivalents for commonly prescribed opioids

Opioid	Conversion factor
Codeine	0.15
Hydrocodone	1
Hydromorphone	4
Morphine	1
Oxycodone	1.5

Data from Centers for Disease Control and Prevention. CDC guideline for prescribing opioids for chronic pain. https://www.cdc.gov/drugoverdose/prescribing/guideline.html. Published August 29, 2017. Accessed February 4, 2019.

MULTIMODAL PAIN CONTROL

Multimodal pain control or "balanced analgesia" relies on several different drugs that act at various places along the pain pathway.[19,24] Adequate pain control postoperatively allows for a more expeditious recovery, allowing for return to activity and work sooner.[19] The use of multimodal pain control can greatly improve overall pain management and decrease opioid consumption.[19] The concept of multimodal postoperative pain control was introduced by Kehlet and Dahl in their landmark article in 1993, yet this notion has been slow to be adopted by many surgeons.[24] Regional anesthesia, liposomal bupivacaine, nonsteroidal anti-inflammatory drugs (NSAIDS), acetaminophen, gabapentin and pregabalin, and hydroxyzine can be used postoperatively to decrease the amount of opioid consumption required for pain control. The authors preferred multimodal pain regimen for foot and ankle surgery is depicted in **Box 1**.

OPIOIDS

Opioids produce analgesia by binding to and activating the opioid receptors in the central and peripheral nervous system, thereby inhibiting release of the neurotransmitter and blocking transmission of the pain signals.[1] Opioids are grouped into 3 categories: natural, semi-synthetic, and synthetic.[1] Natural opioids include morphine and codeine, and semi-synthetic opioids include oxycodone, hydrocodone, and hydromorphone. The synthetic opioids most frequently prescribed include fentanyl and tramadol. The US Food and Drug Administration also recently approved another synthetic opioid that is due on the market soon: Dsuvia, which is 10 times stronger than fentanyl.[1] Common side effects of opioids include itching, urinary retention, constipation, nausea, and vomiting.[8,25] However, it is the side effects of euphoria and dysphoria that make these drugs prone to abuse.[8] Patients can also develop tolerance and opioid-induced hyperesthesia from chronic opioid use.[26] The most concerning side-effect of opioids is respiratory depression, and this is the leading cause of death associated with opioid use.[25] Immediate-release opioids, such as hydrocodone and oxycodone, are the most commonly prescribed following foot and ankle surgery. Extended-release opioids do not, and should not, play a role in acute pain management after foot and ankle surgery and are not recommended by CDC or by AAOS.[11,22]

REGIONAL ANESTHESIA

Foot and ankle surgery lends itself well to regional anesthesia, which can provide improved pain control and decreased opioid use postoperatively.[27] Popliteal nerve blocks and continuous-infusion catheters have been shown to be effective for

---

Box 1
The authors preferred multimodal pain regimen for foot and ankle surgery

Popliteal block or indwelling catheter depending on the complexity of procedure combined with a saphenous block or catheter as indicated.

Gabapentin 600 mg 2 hours preoperatively

Oxycodone 5 mg every 4 to 6 hours as needed for pain, 30 tabs; 42 tabs, depending on the complexity of the procedure

Tylenol 1000 mg every 8 hours (caution in patients with hepatic insufficiency)

Gabapentin 200 mg every 8 hours

Hydroxyzine 25 mg every 8 hours (caution in use of patients older than 65 years)

postoperative pain control.[28] Popliteal nerve blocks can provide up to 24 hours of pain control, and a continuous-infusion catheter can provide up to 72 hours of pain relief.[29] Jarell and colleagues[29] found that combined popliteal and saphenous nerve continuous-infusion catheters provided superior pain control for patients undergoing foot and ankle surgery, especially when there were significant medical procedures performed during the operation.

Ease of obtaining popliteal blocks or infusion nerve catheters varies among institutions. Hegewald and colleagues[30] found an overall success rate of 76.2% for popliteal blocks performed by podiatry residents in patients undergoing foot and ankle surgery. In the same study, they found that popliteal blocks were less successful in younger patients and those with a higher body mass index.[30] Unfortunately, regional anesthesia is not without complications. In a study by Anderson and colleagues,[31] 1014 patients who had foot or ankle surgery underwent a popliteal block and 52 (5%) had neuropathic symptoms that were likely a result of the block. These neuropathic symptoms did not resolve in 7 (0.7%) patients.[31] The authors routinely use regional anesthesia for elective forefoot as well as for rearfoot surgery cases. It is the authors' experience that supplemental intravenous opioids are rarely required in the opioid-naive patient if successful regional anesthesia has been performed.

LIPOSOMAL BUPIVACAINE

In lieu of a popliteal block nerve block, injectable bupivacaine encapsulated within a liposome (EXPAREL) has been formulated for local use at the surgical site allowing a sustained release for over 72 hours.[25] The use of liposomal bupivacaine was first studied in bunion surgery and now has many additional indications.[32] Liposomal bupivacaine has been shown to decrease the amount of opioids consumed after foot surgery.[33] Mulligan and colleagues[34] compared liposomal bupivacaine with continuous popliteal sciatic nerve catheters with ropivacaine in patients who had undergone total ankle arthroplasty, and found liposomal bupivacaine comparable in terms of safety and efficacy. Bupivacaine may be injected immediately before the procedure, or mixed with liposomal bupivacaine, but the ratio of the milligram dose of bupivacaine to EXPAREL must not exceed 1:2.[35] Non-bupivacaine local amide anesthetics, such as lidocaine, may be used 20 minutes before injection with liposomal bupivacaine, but cannot be used again until 96 hours thereafter, otherwise the bupivacaine will be released immediately, possibly leading to cardiac arrest.[34] In addition, liposomal bupivacaine has not been studied in patients under the age of 18 years.[34] The authors recommend fully reading the product insert before use. Liposomal bupivacaine may be beneficial in institutions where regional anesthesia is not readily available.

NONSTEROIDAL ANTI-INFLAMMATORY DRUGS

The mechanism of action of NSAIDs is by the inhibition of 2 cyclooxygenase enzymes, COX-1 and COX-2, thereby decreasing postoperative inflammation and associated pain.[25] Selective COX-2 inhibitors have less gastrointestinal side effects than COX-1, but have possible increased cardiovascular risk.[25] In a study by Daniels and colleagues[36] of postoperative bunionectomy patients, 99 postoperative bunionectomy patients received 25 mg diclofenac soft gel capsules every 4 hours and were compared with 101 patients who received a placebo. In this study, patients receiving diclofenac used less opioid pain medication and had better pain control compared with the placebo group.[36] The use of soft gel capsules is more advantageous postoperatively than other forms because of the rapid absorption and quicker onset.[36] The use of NSAIDS in foot and ankle surgery may be somewhat limited because of the inhibition of bone healing demonstrated in animal models, and the concomitant use of postoperative anticoagulants for deep vein prophylaxis in many cases.[25] A single dose of intravenous ketorolac given immediately postoperatively has been shown to be helpful in patients who have undergone soft tissue procedures. In addition, NSAIDS should be used with caution in any patients with renal insufficiency.[25]

ACETAMINOPHEN

The exact mechanism of action of acetaminophen is unknown, but it is believed to inhibit COX in the central nervous system and affect serotonin activity.[25] Acetaminophen dosed at therapeutic levels, 1 g every 8 hours, can be used to augment opioids. Remy and colleagues[37] studied 265 patients who received morphine by way of a patient-controlled analgesia (PCA) pump along with acetaminophen and compared them with 226 patients who received morphine PCA alone after major surgery. It was shown that patients who received acetaminophen used 20% less morphine.[37] Although several combinations of opioids and acetaminophen are available on the market, the authors prefer to prescribe acetaminophen separately, so that the therapeutic levels of acetaminophen can be reached without increasing the amount of opioids consumed. Acetaminophen is well tolerated by most patients with minimal side effects, but should be used with caution in patients with hepatic insufficiency.[25]

GABAPENTIN AND PREGABALIN

Gabapentin and pregabalin act by blocking calcium channels, thereby inhibiting the transmission of pain in the central and peripheral nervous.[25,38] Although pregabalin is more costly than gabapentin and is considered to be a scheduled drug, it does have a quicker onset of action, which is desirable postoperatively.[25] Buvanendran and colleagues[39] conducted a study of 113 patients after total knee arthroplasty who received 300 mg of pregabalin preoperatively, followed by 150 mg twice daily for 10 days, 75 mg twice daily for 2 days, and 50 mg twice daily for 2 days, and compared the level of pain experienced by the study group with the pain experienced by 115 placebo patients. In their study, patients who received pregabalin had less pain postoperatively and consumed less opioids.[39] In the same study, increased sedation and confusion were reported on the first postoperative day in patients treated with pregabalin.[39]

Several studies support the use of gabapentin as an adjunct both preoperatively and postoperatively in lower extremity surgery.[38] In a study by Clarke and colleagues,[40] of 155 patients undergoing a total knee arthroplasty, 79 patients received a preoperative dose of gabapentin, 600 mg 2 hours before surgery, and then also prescribed gabapentin 200 mg 3 times a day for 4 days postoperatively. In their study, the patients treated with gabapentin had less pain during the first 24 hours compared with the control group.[40] Gabapentin or pregabalin can be helpful adjunctive medications for postoperative pain control but common side effects of both drugs are dizziness and somnolence.[25]

HYDROXYZINE

Antihistamines act by binding to histamine receptors, which are located throughout the body and traditionally are used for allergy relief or to treat gastric reflux.[41] Hydroxyzine is the most well-studied antihistamine for postoperative pain control, but has lost some popularity in recent years.[41] It has been shown to potentiate the analgesic effect of opioids, although the mechanism of action remains speculative.[41,42] Hupert and colleagues[42] found that combining hydroxyzine with morphine provided superior pain control to patients after abdominal surgery compared with morphine alone. Hydroxyzine can also alleviate some of the negative side effects of opioids including itching, nausea, and vomiting.[42] In addition, hydroxyzine has an anxiolytic effect, which can be beneficial postoperatively.[42] Hydroxyzine, however, does induce increased somnolence when combined with opioids compared with opioids alone.[42] Hydroxyzine can also cause respiratory depression and should be used with caution in the elderly.[43]

OPIOID MANAGEMENT IN THE OPIOID-TOLERANT PATIENT

Preoperative communication with a pain management specialist is paramount in an already opioid-tolerant patient, because they will typically require 2 to 3 times more opioids postoperatively than opioid-naive patients.[44] Opioid-tolerant patients are at an increased risk for respiratory depression, and a prescription for rescue naloxone should be considered.[44,45] Pain management for patients on methadone or buprenorphine-naloxone therapy can also be challenging. Patients on methadone therapy should continue their current dose, and additional postoperative opioid pain medication can be prescribed as needed.[44] Communication should take place with the patient's methadone clinic and the patient's dose should be verified.[44] In addition, dividing a patient's total daily methadone dose into 3 times daily can help aid in pain control.[44] Although multiple options exist for the perioperative management of patient's on buprenorphine-naloxone therapy, only one is practical for the podiatric surgeon.[44] With the approval of the patient's pain management specialist, buprenorphine-naloxone should be discontinued 48 hours before surgery.[44] The patient should then be prescribed a postoperative course of opioid pain medication and, when completed, the patient should resume buprenorphine-naloxone.[44] With this option the patient is potentially at risk for withdrawal, although buprenorphine can remain at the receptor site up for up to 5 days after the last dose.[44]

SUMMARY

The United States has had a long history of opioid misuse. Clearly, a change in our pain culture will have to occur for the opioid epidemic to improve. Federal and state laws are evolving in response to the opioid crisis, and establishing more clear guidelines for physicians and patients should follow. Until national guidelines for acute postoperative opioid prescriptions exist, physicians should strive to practice safer opioid prescribing habits. Multimodal pain control is the key to reducing opioid consumption. Prescribing fewer opioids, educating patients on opioid risks, proper disposal of unused medications, and participating in prescription-monitoring programs can help reduce opioid misuse, dependence, and related deaths.

REFERENCES

1. Rosenblum A, Marsch L, Joseph H. Opioids and the treatment of chronic pain: controversies, current status, and future directions. Exp Clin Psychopharmacol 2008;16:405–16.
2. Lawson C. America's 150-year opioid epidemic. New York Times 2018. Available at: https://www.nytimes.com/2018/05/19/opinion/sunday/opioid-epidemic-history.html. Accessed February 10, 2019.

3. Bernard S, Chelminski P, Ives T, et al. Management of pain in the United States-a brief history and implications for the opioid epidemic. Health Serv Insights 2018;11:106.

4. Courtright D. The controlled substances act: how a "big tent" reform became a punitive drug law. Drug Alcohol Depend 2004;76:9–15.

5. Soelberg C, Brown R, Vivier D, et al. The US opioid crisis: current federal and state legal issues. Anesth Analg 2017;125:1675–81.

6. Gross J, Perate A, Elkassabany N. Pain management in trauma in the age of the opioid crisis. Anesthesiol Clin 2019;37:79–91.

7. Jones G, Bruera E, Abdi S, et al. The opioid epidemic in the United States-overview, origins, and potential solutions. Cancer 2018;124:4279–86.

8. Manchikanti L, Singh A. Therapeutic opioids: a ten-Year Perspective on the complexities and complications of the escalating use, abuse, and nonmedical use of opioids. Pain Physician 2008;11:S63–88.

9. Katz J. Drug deaths in America are rising faster than ever. New York Times 2017. Available at: https://www.nytimes.com/interactive/2017/06/05/upshot/opioid-epidemic-drug-overdose-deaths-are-rising-faster-than-ever.html?mtrref=www.google.com. Accessed February 4, 2019.

10. Centers for Disease Control and Prevention. Prescription opioid data. 2018. Available at: https://www.cdc.gov/drugoverdose/data/prescribing.html. Accessed February 4, 2019.

11. American Academy of Orthopaedic Surgeons. Opioid use, misuse, and abuse in orthopaedic practice. 2011. Available at: https://www.aaos.org/uploadedFiles/PreProduction/About/Opinion_Statements/advistmt/1045%20Opioid%20Use,%20Misuse,%20and%20Abuse%20in%20Practice.pdf.

12. Merrill H, Dean D, Mottla J, et al. Opioid consumption following foot and ankle surgery. Foot Ankle Int 2018;39:649–56.

13. Lindenhovious A, Helmerhorts G, Schnellen A. Differences in prescription of narcotic pain medication after operative treatment of hip and ankle fractures in the United States and The Netherlands. J Trauma 2009;67:160–4.

14. Chou L, Wagner D, Witten D, et al. Postoperative pain following foot and ankle surgery: a prospective study. Foot Ankle Int 2008;29:1063–8.

15. Saini S, McDonald E, Shakked R, et al. Prospective evaluation of utilization patterns and prescribing guidelines of in-depth opioid consumption following orthopedic foot and ankle surgery. Foot Ankle Int 2018;39:1257–65.

16. Ghoneim M, O'Hara M. Depression and postoperative complications: an overview. BMC Surg 2016;16:1–10.

17. Devin C, Lee D, Armaghani S, et al. Approach to pain management in chronic opioid users undergoing orthopaedic surgery. J Am Acad Orthop Surg 2014; 22(10):614–22.

18. Gupta A, Kumar K, Roberts M, et al. Pain management after outpatient foot and ankle surgery. Foot Ankle Int 2018;39:149–54.

19. Parvizi J, Miller A, Gandhi K. Multimodal pain management after total joint arthroplasty. J Bone Joint Surg Am 2011;93:1075–84.

20. Zgierska A, Rabago D, Miller M. Impact of patient satisfaction ratings on physicians and clinical care. Patient Prefer Adherence 2014;8:437–46.

21. Dyer O. US doctor is shot dead after refusing to prescribe opioids. BMJ 2017; 358:j3724.

22. Centers for Disease Control and Prevention. CDC guideline for prescribing opioids for chronic pain. 2017. Available at: https://www.cdc.gov/drugoverdose/prescribing/guideline.html. Accessed February 4, 2019.

23. Washington State Department of Health. Washington state opioid prescribing requirements. 2018. Available at: https://www.doh.wa.gov/Portals/1/Documents/9220/631076-PrescriberHandout-Podiatry.pdf. Accessed February 10, 2019.

24. Kehlet H, Dahl J. The value of "multimodal" or "balanced analgesia" in postoperative pain treatment. Anesth Analg 1993;77:1048–55.

25. Khoring J, Orgain N. Multimodal analgesia in foot and ankle surgery. Orthop Clin North Am 2017;48:495–505.

26. Coluzzi F, Bifulco F, Cuomo A, et al. The challenge of perioperative pain management in opioid-tolerant patients. Ther Clin Risk Manag 2017;13:1163–73.

27. Vadivelu N, Kai A, Maslin B, et al. Role of regional anesthesia in foot and ankle surgery. Foot Ankle Spec 2015;8:212–9.

28. Fraser T, Doty J. Peripheral nerve blocks in foot and ankle surgery. Orthop Clin North Am 2017;48:507–15.

29. Jarrell K, McDonald E, Shakked R, et al. Combined popliteal catheter with single-injection vs continuous-infusion saphenous nerve block for foot and ankle surgery. Foot Ankle Int 2018;39:332–7.

30. Hegewald K, McCann K, Elizaga A, et al. Popliteal blocks for foot and ankle surgery: success rate and contributing factors. J Foot Ankle Surg 2014;53:176–8.

31. Anderson J, Bohay D, Maskill J, et al. Complications after popliteal block for foot and ankle surgery. Foot Ankle Int 2015;36:1138–43.

32. Golf M, Daniels S, Onel E. A phase 3, randomized, placebo-controlled trial of depofoam® bupivacaine (extended-release bupivacaine local analgesic) in bunionectomy. Adv Ther 2011;28:776–88.

33. Robbins J, Green C, Parekh S. Liposomal bupivacaine in forefoot surgery. Foot Ankle Int 2015;36:503–7.

34. Mulligan R, Morash J, DeOrio J, et al. Liposomal bupivacaine versus continuous popliteal sciatic nerve block in total ankle arthroplasty. Foot Ankle Int 2017;38:1222–8.

35. Pacira Pharmaceuticals. EXPAREL (bupivacaine liposome injectable suspension). San Diego (CA): Pacira Pharmaceuticals; 2018 [package insert].

36. Daniels S, Baum D, Clark F, et al. Diclofenac potassium liquid-filled soft gelatin capsules for the treatment of postbunionectomy pain. Curr Med Res Opin 2010;26:2375–84.

37. Remy C, Marret R, Bonnet F. Effects of acetaminophen on morphine side effects and consumption after major surgery: meta analysis of randomized controlled trials. Br J Anaesth 2005;94:505–13.

38. Crisologo P, Monson E, Atway S. Gabapentin as an adjunct to standard postoperative pain management protocol in lower extremity surgery. J Foot Ankle Surg 2018;57:781–4.

39. Buvanendran A, Kroin J, Della Valle C, et al. Perioperative oral pregabalin reduces chronic pain after total knee arthroplasty: a prospective, randomized, controlled trial. Anesth Analg 2010;110:199–207.

40. Clarke H, Pereira S, Kennedy D, et al. Gabapentin decreases morphine consumption and improves functional recovery following total knee arthroplasty. Pain Res Manag 2009;14:217–22.

41. Rumore M, Schlichting D. Clinical efficacy of antihistamines as analgesics. Pain 1986;25:7–22.

42. Hupert C, Yacoub M, Turgeon L. Effect of hydroxyzine on morphine analgesia for the treatment of postoperative pain. Anesth Analg 1980;59:690–6.

43. Glazier H. Potentiation of pain relief with hydroxyzine: a therapeutic myth? Annuals Pharmacother 1990;24:485–8.

44. Vaghari B, Baratta J, Gandi K. Perioperative approach to patients with opioid abuse and tolerance. Anesthesiology News 2013;June. Available at: https://www.anesthesiologynews.com/download/Opioid_AN0613_WM.pdf. Accessed February 6, 2019.

45. Teckchandani S, Barad M. Treatment strategies for the opioid-dependent patient. Curr Pain Headache Rep 2017;45:1–9.

Women in Podiatry and Medicine

Brittany A. Brower, DPM[a],*, Meagan M. Jennings, DPM[b],
Michelle L. Butterworth, DPM[c], Mary E. Crawford, DPM[d]

KEYWORDS

- Physicians • Women physicians • Podiatry • Gender bias • Publications
- Academic medicine • Discrimination • Feminization of medicine

KEY POINTS

- The feminization of medicine is changing the medical community, although female physicians continue to face prejudice and barriers to closing the gender gap.
- Female physicians continue to have lower academic standings and fewer publications, receive less awards/grants, are underrepresented in leadership positions, have a lower incidence of pursuing surgical specialties, and receive lower compensation.
- Burnout, gender discrimination, and sexual harassment are prevalent throughout medicine and a detriment to the profession.
- Increased awareness with the goal to implement change is key to achieving gender equity.

INTRODUCTION

Over the past 170 years, the role of female physicians has undoubtedly advanced among western medicine.[1] Historically, medicine has been a male-dominated field with women serving primarily as nurses, midwives, healers, and caretakers.[2] The Passage of Title IX of the Higher Educational Act served as a major turning point in the medical field, as it prohibited discrimination based on sex in any federally funded education program or activity, including postgraduate programs. Within 2 years, the proportion of women entering US medical schools doubled, and by 2012, women made up one-third of all physicians.[3] Today they outnumber men in US medical schools (50.7%).[4] Recently, women have been able to crack through the glass ceiling, making

---

Disclosure Information: The authors have nothing to disclose.
[a] John Peter Smith Hospital, 1500 South Main Street, Fort Worth, TX 76104, USA; [b] Silicon Valley Foot & Ankle Reconstructive Surgery Fellowship, Palo Alto Medical Foundation, 701 E. El Camino Real South Wing, Mountain View, CA 94040, USA; [c] Williamsburg Regional Hospital, 500 Thurgood Marshall Hwy, Suite B, Kingstree, SC 29556, USA; [d] Providence Regional Medical Center, Private Practice at the Ankle & Foot Clinics Northwest, 3131 Nassaeu Street Suite 101, Everett, WA 98291, USA
* Corresponding author. 1418 E Millbrook Road, Raleigh, NC 27609.
E-mail address: brittanybrower6@gmail.com

Clin Podiatr Med Surg 36 (2019) 707–716
https://doi.org/10.1016/j.cpm.2019.06.010
0891-8422/19/© 2019 Elsevier Inc. All rights reserved.

strides toward closing the gender gap.[2] In April 2017 the #ILookLikeASurgeon media campaign gained national recognition in hopes to promote diversity in surgical fields and open peoples' minds to the idea that women can be surgeons or anything else they desire.[5] This campaign, along with others such as #HeforShe and #AsAWomen, all symbolize how important and timely this topic is, as now is the time for women to be recognized as leaders in their field.

Podiatric female physicians have paralleled the numerical increase seen in general medicine. From 1969 to 2015, the percentage of women in podiatry has increased from 1% to 39% with a maximum increase of 47% in 2004 and 2005.[6]

Despite the feminization of medicine, female physicians continue to face prejudice and barriers to their advancement. Female physicians have lower reported academic standings and fewer publications, receive less awards, are underrepresented in leadership positions, have a lower incidence of pursuing surgical specialties, receive lower compensation, and experience an increased rate of burnout, gender discrimination, and sexual harassment[7–17] (Brower BA, Butterworth ML, Crawford ME, et al. The Podiatric Medical Profession: A Gender Comparison. Submitted for Publication).

CONTENT

The cause of female underrepresentation in medicine is unknown and likely multifactorial. There has been minimal published research on the gender gap in podiatric medicine and surgery; therefore causation can only be speculated.

So how do we achieve gender equity? Many have speculated that with time, the gap will passively close as more women enter this profession. However, the current number of female applicants to the podiatric profession has plateaued over the past 10 years (Brower BA, Butterworth ML, Crawford ME, et al. The Podiatric Medical Profession: A Gender Comparison. Submitted for Publication). Therefore, despite the increasing number of women in medicine, there continues to be a lack of female representation in surgical specialties. According to the American Medical Association (AMA), only 19.2% of women are surgeons.[18] The shortage of women in male-dominated surgical specialties has been attributed to limited clinical exposure during medical school, difficulty in achieving a good work/life balance, organizational tolerance for sexually harassing behavior, and lack of strong female mentorship.[12,19,20]

EMPLOYMENT

The lack of a healthy work/life balance is frequently discussed in the literature as a common denominator for why women avoid surgical specialties. Longer nonflexible work hours, decreased availability of part-time opportunities, spousal career, and insufficient home support may all contribute to the underlying cause. Our society has progressed away from traditional gender roles, although it seems that for some, male careers continue to outrank female careers, when comparing spousal professions (Brower BA, Butterworth ML, Crawford ME, et al. The Podiatric Medical Profession: A Gender Comparison. Submitted for Publication). In addition, increased home support, seen more commonly with male physicians, may provide those individuals with more time and flexibility to advance in their career[7] (Brower BA, Butterworth ML, Crawford ME, et al. The Podiatric Medical Profession: A Gender Comparison. Submitted for Publication).

Nationally, female physicians are reported to work part-time 22% of the time and male physicians 12%.[21] Podiatric female physicians work part-time 18.9% of the time compared with 15.4% by men (Brower BA, Butterworth ML, Crawford ME, et al. The Podiatric Medical Profession: A Gender Comparison. Submitted for

Publication). Part-time employment opportunities have been depicted as a beneficial option for those individuals seeking a work-life balance, although many job positions may not offer this type of flexibility.[21]

Academic Positions

The Association of American Medical Colleges (AAMC) revealed that women are underrepresented in academic medicine. Women in the academic setting make up 34% of the associate professors, 21% of the full professors, 15% of the department chairs, and 16% of the deans.[22] The lack of women in leadership positions is paralleled in the podiatric medicine and surgery community. Women are underrepresented as lecturers at national meetings, members of board committees, and editors; have lower academic rankings; are involved in less research activities/produce less publications; and on average are less Reconstructive Rearfoot/Ankle (RRA) board qualified/certified compared with male counterparts (Brower BA, Butterworth ML, Crawford ME, et al. The Podiatric Medical Profession: A Gender Comparison. Submitted for Publication).

Mentorship plays a large role in career advancement. Those individuals with mentors spend more time on research, publish more articles, feel more confident, and are overall more satisfied with their careers compared with those without mentors.[23] Both genders can be very effective mentors, although when men are the only source of mentorship for women, it may be difficult for them to identify with the pressures women confront in the field of medicine. In addition, men may be apprehensive toward mentoring women, as there is a higher potential for misunderstandings to occur between genders.[7]

There are currently less female mentors available in the academic setting, with an increased female desire for same-sex mentors (Brower BA, Butterworth ML, Crawford ME, et al. The Podiatric Medical Profession: A Gender Comparison. Submitted for Publication).[22] Unfortunately, with a lack of women in leadership positions throughout medicine, this need cannot be easily fulfilled. Seeing other women lead well-balanced work-life schedules while also advancing their academic career may benefit women in junior positions to feel more comfortable pursing a similar path.[7,23,24]

Male physicians have a substantially higher number of publications[8] (Brower BA, Butterworth ML, Crawford ME, et al. The Podiatric Medical Profession: A Gender Comparison. Submitted for Publication). Male podiatric physicians publish 5 times more than female podiatric physicians do (Brower BA, Butterworth ML, Crawford ME, et al. The Podiatric Medical Profession: A Gender Comparison. Submitted for Publication). The literature has attributed this to an increased number of grants provided to men and better access to mentors.[8,25] Underrepresentation of women as recipients of grants and awards occurs across many subspecialties and is associated with exclusively male-dominated award committees.[9,26,27] Unfortunately, grants provided to women through organizations such as American College of Foot and Ankle Surgeons have been limited (Brower BA, Butterworth ML, Crawford ME, et al. The Podiatric Medical Profession: A Gender Comparison. Submitted for Publication).

Podiatric Medicine and Surgery

When evaluating podiatric medicine and surgery by subspecialties, surgery is a main focus for both genders, although women spend more time in a clinical setting compared with men (Brower BA, Butterworth ML, Crawford ME, et al. The Podiatric Medical Profession: A Gender Comparison. Submitted for Publication). This could be secondary to differences between gender practicing and communication styles.[28] Women cultivate a collaborative relationship with the patient through encouragement and empathy. They spend more time with the patient in order to feel as though they have provided the patient with quality care.[25,28–30] Conversely, male physicians spend less time with patients, tend to speak in an authoritative manner, and interrupt more often, giving off a distant form of communication.[28–30]

DISCRIMINATION AND HARASSMENT

The time periods 2017 and 2018, "The Year of the Women," were defining years for women's issues with the #MeToo and #TimesUp movements. Despite this momentum, the health care system continues to lag behind.[20,31,32] Sexual harassment and gender discrimination have a significant prevalence in high-powered fields with a hierarchical system and in male-dominated specialties, specifically those with long hours and high-stress environments in an operating room type culture.[15,33–35]

The National Academies of Sciences, Engineering, and Medicine documented this culture in a groundbreaking report released in 2018. This report opened the public's eyes to the shockingly high prevalence of harassment, encouraging national organizations to initiate change. Subsequently, statements by the AAMC, AMA, and National Institute of Health were produced condemning sexual harassment. According to the report, 40% of medical students reported sexual harassment in academic medicine, which almost doubled that of other science and engineering specialties, with most of the perpetrators being faculty or staff. This causes a decline in job satisfaction, burnout, increased stress, poor performance, withdrawal from organizations, and loss of talent.[20] The AAMC's 2017 Medical School Graduation Questionnaire reported only 21% of students who experienced a form of harassment reported it.[36]

There are very few studies in the literature evaluating gender discrimination and sexual harassment in medicine, let alone in the podiatric medicine and surgery community. A meta-analysis evaluating the prevalence of harassment in residency was performed among 11,193 residents. About 63.4% reported experiencing harassment, with gender discrimination and verbal abuse as the most common forms.[37] A national survey on US women medical doctors found 47.7% experienced gender discrimination and 36.9% sexual harassment. The majority was seen within a training environment and mostly in male-dominated fields.[15] Another survey evaluating female general surgeons measured perceptions and impact of gender-based discrimination in medical school, residency training, and surgical practice. Eighty-seven percent experienced gender-based discrimination in medical school, 88% in residency, and 91% in practice.[17] Comparatively, a national survey of the general public reported 42% of the general population experienced gender discrimination and 22% sexual harassment.[16]

A higher percentage of harassment occurs in a training environment, and this statement holds true among the podiatric medicine and surgery community as well.[15,17,37] A recent study evaluated harassment in podiatric residencies across the United States and found 82% of women and 41% of men experienced sexist hostility, 55% of women and 32% of men experienced sexual hostility, and 26% of women and 7% of men experienced unwanted sexual attention. The highest reported perpetrators of harassment were residency directors or attendings at 38%. Thirty-four percent of residents were unaware if their program had an established reporting protocol, and 35% felt uncomfortable reporting harassment.[38]

Another survey evaluated gender discrimination and sexual harassment among the podiatric medicine and surgery community. Seventy-three percent of women and 5.7% of men reported experiencing gender discrimination (**Fig. 1**), and 41.5% of women and 5% of men reported experiencing sexual harassment (**Fig. 2**). The main culprits for both types of harassment were superiors for women and patients for men. The most significant amount of harassment occurred in states with podiatric

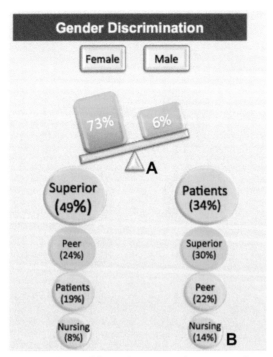

Fig. 1. (*A*) Percentage data obtained from the survey of women and men who have experienced gender discrimination within the podiatry profession. (*B*) Relationship to the offender.

medical schools and those with an increased amount of residency programs. These states included California, New York, Florida, Illinois, Ohio, Pennsylvania, New Jersey, Washington, Georgia, Arizona, and Michigan (Brower BA, Butterworth ML, Crawford ME, et al. The Podiatric Medical Profession: A Gender Comparison. Submitted for Publication).

The podiatric medical community's incidence of harassment is comparable to the rate reported among the general surgery community.[17] This is likely due to a similar high-stress surgical environment, in a historically male-dominated field based on hierarchy.[35] With men being the dominate form of leadership at many institutions and reported as the most common source of harassment, this negative culture may continue to be toxic to the academic medicine environment if change is not implemented. To create change, leaders needs to make explicit statements about sexual harassment, including the consequences that will result for perpetrators who violate the harassment policies.[39]

COMPENSATION

Despite the medical field progressing over the past century, there continues to be a significant wage gap. Female physicians were reported to make almost $20,000 less per year than male physicians, and women in surgical subspecialties made roughly $44,000 less per year compared with men.[13,31] These numbers are after adjusting for age, experience, specialty, faculty rank, and measures of research productivity and clinical revenue. This wage gap is not caused by fewer hours worked or difference in performance.[13,31] In fact, another study found that female physicians

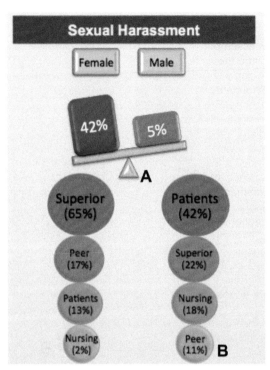

Fig. 2. (*A*) Percentage data obtained from the survey of women and men who have experienced sexual harassment within the podiatry profession. (*B*) Relationship to the offender.

have better outcomes than those of male doctors. If men provided the same quality care as women, they could save an additional 32,000 lives per year.[40] This is largely disconcerting, especially now that women make up most of the medical students.[4]

Podiatric medicine and surgery physician salaries were evaluated by Podiatry Management's Annual Survey (2018), which reported that women only earn 68% of what their male colleagues do. This study also stated that board-certified podiatric physicians earned higher incomes.[14]

PHYSICIAN BURNOUT

Another prominent issue by which all medical specialties have been negatively affected is physician burnout. It affects nearly half (44%) of all practicing physicians and seems to be escalating. According to Medscape's 2019 report, 50% of female doctors and 39% of male doctors reported burnout. The report suggested that women are more likely to admit to psychological problems and seek help; therefore, they acknowledge burnout more often compared with men.[41] Female physicians' higher burnout rate has been associated with feelings of less control over their work, lower mean income, additional hours worked per week, communication style, imposter syndrome/stereotype perception, gendered expectations, sexual harassment/gender bias, and having young children in conjunction with minimal home support.[20,25,42] In addition, many female surgeons (39%) consider changing their career once they become pregnant during training due to concerns regarding work hours and inadequate maternity leave packages.[43]

DISCUSSION

There is a common assumption that as the number of women in medicine increases, more women will climb the academic ladder, harassment and gender bias will dissipate, and the wage gap will close. The medical community has made strides toward gender equality, although continues to lag behind fortune 500 companies, academic science, and engineering (Brower BA, Butterworth ML, Crawford ME, et al. The Podiatric Medical Profession: A Gender Comparison. Submitted for Publication).[20,27]

Most female podiatric physicians have lower academic standings and fewer publications, receive less awards/grants, are underrepresented in leadership positions, work fewer hours, have a lower incidence of RRA certifications, are less satisfied in their careers, experience increased rates of harassment, and report higher stress levels compared with men (Brower BA, Butterworth ML, Crawford ME, et al. The Podiatric Medical Profession: A Gender Comparison. Submitted for Publication).

Encouraging institutions to recruit strong female physicians is in the best interest of academic centers, although it needs to happen as an institutional transformation.[10] This will create a positive downstream effect for future women in medicine. Fortune 500 companies have been faster than academia to institute such measures. They have benefited through increased overall performance and financial advancement.[10,44]

Fortunately, major academic centers have taken steps toward change. The Mayo Clinic is well known for its advancement of women. They have nearly doubled the number of women in leadership positions since 2010, and in 2014, 70 women were promoted to either associate or full professor, which more than quadruples the number a decade prior.

The University of Pennsylvania has a program called "FOCUS on Health and Leadership for Women" designed to improve the recruitment, retention, advancement, and leadership of women faculty. It also serves to promote education and research in women's health and leadership. This program has one of the strongest budget lines of any Women in Medicine program in the United States. Additionally, Yale medicine's new Department of Surgery Chair is a female oncology surgeon making groundbreaking changes in a historically male-dominated specialty.[39] These institutions have created a huge culture shift, paving the way for female physicians.

To encourage change among the podiatric medicine and surgery community, both the scientific and professional societies should help increase awareness to promote the following:

- Equal opportunity to both genders in academic medicine, leadership positions, and representation at national conferences
- Eliminate harassment
- Advocate for transparency of salaries
- Recognize and select the most qualified candidates based on merit

In addition, discrimination and reverse discrimination should be prevented in order to avoid diluting the quality of representation. With the feminization of medicine, increasing awareness of the gender gap is vital to the enhancement of our profession.

REFERENCES

1. Ward L. Female Faculty in male-dominated fields: law, medicine, and engineering. New Dir High Educ 2008;(143):63–72.

2. Livingston RS. Women in medicine: past, present, & future. Carbondale (IL): Southern Illinois University Carbondale; 2015. Honors Theses. Paper 390.

3. Perry S. How Title IX helped make women's dreams of becoming doctors a reality. Minnesota Post 2017. Available at: https://www.minnpost.com/second-opinion/2017/01/how-title-ix-helped-make-womens-dreams-becoming-doctors-reality/. Accessed March 19, 2019.

4. Press Release. More women than men enrolled in U.S. Medical Schools in 2017. AAMC News 2017. Available at: https://news.aamc.org/press-releases/article/applicant-enrollment-2017/. Accessed March 22, 2019.

5. Ault A. #ilooklikeasurgeon gets new boost from New Yorker cover. Medscape 2017. Available at: https://www.medscape.com/viewarticle/878843/. Accessed March 21, 2019.

6. American Association of Colleges of Podiatric Medicine. Statistics 2016. Available at: https://www.aacpm.org/statistics/. Accessed March 22, 2019.

7. Yedidia MJ, Bickel J. Why aren't there more women leaders in academic medicine? The views of clinical department chairs. Acad Med 2001;76:453–65.

8. Fridner A, Norell A, Akesson F, et al. Possible reasons why female physicians publish fewer scientific articles than male physicians-a cross-sectional study. BMC Med Educ 2015;15:67.

9. Silver JK, Bhatnagar S, Blauwet CA, et al. Female physicians are underrepresented in recognition awards from the American Academy of Physical Medicine and Rehabilitation. PM R 2017;9(10):976–84.

10. Bickel J, Wara D, Atkinson BF, et al. Increasing women's leadership in academic medicine: report of the AAMC project implementation committee. Acad Med 2002;77(10):1043–61.

11. Gargiulo DA, Hyman NH, Herbert JC. Women in surgery. Arch Surg 2006;141:405–8.

12. Lewis VO, Scherl SA, Connor MIO. American Orthopaedic Association critical issues. Women in Orthopaedics — way behind the number curve. J Bone Joint Surg 2012;30:1–7.

13. Jena AB, Olenski AR, Blumenthal DM. Sex differences in physician salary in US public medical schools. JAMA Intern Med 2016;176(9):1294–304.

14. Donoghue SK. Podiatry management 35th annual survey: boosting the bottom line. Podiatry Management 2018;83–126.

15. Frank E, Brogan D, Schiffman M. Prevalence and correlates of harassment among US women physicians. Arch Intern Med 1998;158(4):352–8.

16. Parker K, Funk C, Pew Research Center. Gender discrimination comes in many forms for today's working women 2017. Available at: http://www.pewresearch.org/fact-tank/2017/12/14/gender-discrimination-comes-in-many-forms-for-todays-working-women/. Accessed March 22, 2019.

17. Bruce AN, Battista A, Plankey MW, et al. Perceptions of gender-based discrimination during surgical training and practice. Med Educ Online 2015;20(0):1–10.

18. Wolfe L. Statistics of the number of women surgeons in the United States. The balance careers 2018. Available at: https://www.thebalancecareers.com/number-of-women-surgeons-in-the-us-3972900. Accessed March 21, 2019.

19. Hill JF, Yule A, Zurakowski D, et al. Residents' perceptions of sex diversity in orthopaedic surgery. J Bone Joint Surg Am 2013;95(144):1–6.

20. National Academies of Sciences. Engineering, and Medicine. Sexual harassment of women: climate, culture, and consequences in academic sciences, engineering, and medicine. Washington, DC: National Academies Press; 2018.

21. Higgins C, Duxbury L, Johnson K. Part-time work for women: does it really help balance work and family? Hum Resour Manage 2000;39(1):17–32.

22. The State of Women in Academic Medicine. The pipeline and pathways to leadership. Washington, DC: AAMC; 2014. Available at: https://members.aamc.org/eweb/upload/The%20State%20of%20Women%20in%20Academic%20Medicine%202013-2014%20FINAL.pdf/. Accessed March 23, 2019.
23. Levinson W, Kaufman K, Clark B, et al. Mentors and role models for women in academic medicine. West J Med 1991;154:423–6.
24. Levinson W, Tolle SW, Lewis C. Women in academic medicine: combining career and family. N Engl J Med 1989;321:1511–7.
25. McMurray JE, Linzer M, Konrad TR, et al. The work lives of women physicians. Results from the physician work live study. J Gen Intern Med 2000;15:372–80.
26. Recognizing the achievements of women in science, technology, engineering, mathematics, and medicine. Raise Project 2018. Available at: http://www.raiseproject.org/results.php. Accessed March 22, 2019.
27. Lincoln AE, Pincus S, Koster JB, et al. The Matilda effect in science: awards and prizes in the US, 1990s and 2000s. Soc Stud Sci 2012;42:307–20.
28. Levinson W, Lurie N. When most doctors are women: what lies ahead? Ann Intern Med 2004;141:471–4.
29. Kilminster S, Downes J, Gough B, et al. Women in medicine – is there a problem? A literature review of the changing gender composition, structures and occupational cultures in medicine. Med Educ 2007;41:39–49.
30. Roter DL, Hall JA, Aoki Y. Physician gender effects in medical communication: a meta-analytic review. J Am Med Assoc 2002;288:756–64.
31. Kane L. Medscape physician compensation report 2018 2018. Available at: https://www.medscape.com/slideshow/2018-compensation-overview-6009667?src=wnl_physrep_180425_mscpmrk_comp2018_rm&uac=199803SZ&impID=1616384&faf=1/. Accessed March 22, 2019.
32. Salam M. 2018: year of the woman in 5 powerful quotes. The New York Times 2018. Available at: https://www.nytimes.com/2018/12/28/us/women-2018-biggest-stories-me-too.html. Accessed March 19, 2019.
33. Walton MM. Sexual equality, discrimination and harassment in medicine: it's time to act. Med J Aust 2015;203(4):167–9.
34. Crebbin W, Campbell F, Hillis DA, et al. Prevalence of bullying, discrimination and sexual harassment in surgery in Australasia. ANZ J Surg 2015;85(12):905–9.
35. Bickel J. Women in medical education-A status report. N Engl J Med 1988;319:1579–84.
36. Medical School Graduation Questionnaire. Association of American Medical Colleges. Available at: https://www.aamc.org/download/481784/data/2017gqallschoolssummaryreport.pdf. Accessed March 22, 2019.
37. Fnais N, Soobiah C, Chen MH, et al. Harassment and discrimination in medical training: a systematic review and meta-analysis. Acad Med 2014;89(5):817–27.
38. Ang J, Schneider HP. Harassment in Residency: An Anonymous Survey of Podiatric Residents [Poster]. Exhibited at: ACFAS New Orleans Conference Poster Competition. New Orleans, LA, February 14, 2019.
39. Paturel A. Sexual harassment in medicine. AAMC News 2019. Available at: https://news.aamc.org/diversity/article/sexual-harassment-medicine/. Accessed March 22, 2019.
40. Tsugawa Y, Jena AB, Figueroa JF, et al. Comparison of hospital mortality and readmission rates for Medicare patients treated by male vs. female physicians. JAMA Intern Med 2017;177(2):206–13.

41. National physician burnout, depression & suicide report 2019. Medscape. Available at: https://www.medscape.com/slideshow/2019-lifestyle-burnout-depression-6011056/. Accessed March 23, 2019.

42. Dahlke AR, Johnson JK, Greenberg CC, et al. Gender differences in utilization of duty-hour regulations, aspects of burnout, and psychological well-being among general surgery residents in the United States. Ann Surg 2018;268(2):204–11.

43. Rangel EL, Smink DS, Castillo-Angeles M, et al. Pregnancy and motherhood during surgical training. JAMA Surg 2018;153(7):644–52.

44. Adler R. Women in the executive suite correlate to high profits. Harv Bus Rev 2001;79:3.

UNITED STATES POSTAL SERVICE® Statement of Ownership, Management, and Circulation
(All Periodicals Publications Except Requester Publications)

1. Publication Title	2. Publication Number	3. Filing Date
CLINICS IN PODIATRIC MEDICINE & SURGERY	000 – 707	9/18/2019

4. Issue Frequency	5. Number of Issues Published Annually	6. Annual Subscription Price
JAN, APR, JUL, OCT	4	$304.00

7. Complete Mailing Address of Known Office of Publication (Not printer) (Street, city, county, state, and ZIP+4®)

ELSEVIER INC.
230 Park Avenue, Suite 800
New York, NY 10169

Contact Person: STEPHEN R. BUSHING
Telephone (include area code): 215-239-3688

8. Complete Mailing Address of Headquarters or General Business Office of Publisher (Not printer)

ELSEVIER INC.
230 Park Avenue, Suite 800
New York, NY 10169

9. Full Names and Complete Mailing Addresses of Publisher, Editor, and Managing Editor (Do not leave blank)

Publisher (Name and complete mailing address)
TAYLOR BALL, ELSEVIER INC.
1600 JOHN F KENNEDY BLVD. SUITE 1800
PHILADELPHIA, PA 19103-2899

Editor (Name and complete mailing address)
LAUREN BOYLE, ELSEVIER INC.
1600 JOHN F KENNEDY BLVD. SUITE 1800
PHILADELPHIA, PA 19103-2899

Managing Editor (Name and complete mailing address)
PATRICK MANLEY, ELSEVIER INC.
1600 JOHN F KENNEDY BLVD. SUITE 1800
PHILADELPHIA, PA 19103-2899

10. Owner (Do not leave blank. If the publication is owned by a corporation, give the name and address of the corporation immediately followed by the names and addresses of all stockholders owning or holding 1 percent or more of the total amount of stock. If not owned by a corporation, give the names and addresses of the individual owners. If owned by a partnership or other unincorporated firm, give its name and address as well as those of each individual owner. If the publication is published by a nonprofit organization, give its name and address.)

Full Name	Complete Mailing Address
WHOLLY OWNED SUBSIDIARY OF REED/ELSEVIER, US HOLDINGS	1600 JOHN F KENNEDY BLVD. SUITE 1800 PHILADELPHIA, PA 19103-2899

11. Known Bondholders, Mortgagees, and Other Security Holders Owning or Holding 1 Percent or More of Total Amount of Bonds, Mortgages, or Other Securities. If none, check box ▶ ☐ None

Full Name	Complete Mailing Address
N/A	

12. Tax Status (For completion by nonprofit organizations authorized to mail at nonprofit rates) (Check one)
The purpose, function, and nonprofit status of this organization and the exempt status for federal income tax purposes:
☒ Has Not Changed During Preceding 12 Months
☐ Has Changed During Preceding 12 Months (Publisher must submit explanation of change with this statement)

PS Form 3526, July 2014 (Page 1 of 4 (see instructions page 4)) PSN: 7530-01-000-9931 PRIVACY NOTICE: See our privacy policy on www.usps.com.

---

13. Publication Title	14. Issue Date for Circulation Data Below
CLINICS IN PODIATRIC MEDICINE & SURGERY	JULY 2019

15. Extent and Nature of Circulation		Average No. Copies Each Issue During Preceding 12 Months	No. Copies of Single Issue Published Nearest to Filing Date
a. Total Number of Copies (Net press run)		160	174
b. Paid Circulation (By Mail and Outside the Mail)	(1) Mailed Outside-County Paid Subscriptions Stated on PS Form 3541 (include paid distribution above nominal rate, advertiser's proof copies, and exchange copies)	95	108
	(2) Mailed In-County Paid Subscriptions Stated on PS Form 3541 (include paid distribution above nominal rate, advertiser's proof copies, and exchange copies)	0	0
	(3) Paid Distribution Outside the Mails Including Sales Through Dealers and Carriers, Street Vendors, Counter Sales, and Other Paid Distribution Outside USPS®	11	14
	(4) Paid Distribution by Other Classes of Mail Through the USPS (e.g., First-Class Mail®)	0	0
c. Total Paid Distribution (Sum of 15b (1), (2), (3), and (4))	▶	106	122
d. Free or Nominal Rate Distribution (By Mail and Outside the Mail)	(1) Free or Nominal Rate Outside-County Copies included on PS Form 3541	43	36
	(2) Free or Nominal Rate In-County Copies Included on PS Form 3541	0	0
	(3) Free or Nominal Rate Copies Mailed at Other Classes Through the USPS (e.g., First-Class Mail)	0	0
	(4) Free or Nominal Rate Distribution Outside the Mail (Carriers or other means)	0	0
e. Total Free or Nominal Rate Distribution (Sum of 15d (1), (2), (3) and (4))	▶	43	36
f. Total Distribution (Sum of 15c and 15e)	▶	149	158
g. Copies not Distributed (See Instructions to Publishers #4 (page #3))	▶	11	16
h. Total (Sum of 15f and g)	▶	160	174
i. Percent Paid (15c divided by 15f times 100)	▶	71.14%	77.22%

* If you are claiming electronic copies, go to line 16 on page 3. If you are not claiming electronic copies, skip to line 17 on page 3.

16. Electronic Copy Circulation		Average No. Copies Each Issue During Preceding 12 Months	No. Copies of Single Issue Published Nearest to Filing Date
a. Paid Electronic Copies	▶		
b. Total Paid Print Copies (Line 15c) + Paid Electronic Copies (Line 16a)	▶		
c. Total Print Distribution (Line 15f) + Paid Electronic Copies (Line 16a)	▶		
d. Percent Paid (Both Print & Electronic Copies) (16b divided by 16c × 100)	▶		

☒ I certify that 50% of all my distributed copies (electronic and print) are paid above a nominal price.

17. Publication of Statement of Ownership

☒ If the publication is a general publication, publication of this statement is required. Will be printed in the OCTOBER 2019 issue of this publication. ☐ Publication not required.

18. Signature and Title of Editor, Publisher, Business Manager, or Owner

STEPHEN R. BUSHING - INVENTORY DISTRIBUTION CONTROL MANAGER

Stephen R. Bushing Date 9/18/2019

I certify that all information furnished on this form is true and complete. I understand that anyone who furnishes false or misleading information on this form or who omits material or information requested on the form may be subject to criminal sanctions (including fines and imprisonment) and/or civil sanctions (including civil penalties).

PS Form 3526, July 2014 (Page 3 of 4) PRIVACY NOTICE: See our privacy policy on www.usps.com.

Moving?

Make sure your subscription moves with you!

To notify us of your new address, find your **Clinics Account Number** (located on your mailing label above your name), and contact customer service at:

Email: journalscustomerservice-usa@elsevier.com

800-654-2452 (subscribers in the U.S. & Canada)
314-447-8871 (subscribers outside of the U.S. & Canada)

Fax number: 314-447-8029

Elsevier Health Sciences Division
Subscription Customer Service
3251 Riverport Lane
Maryland Heights, MO 63043

*To ensure uninterrupted delivery of your subscription, please notify us at least 4 weeks in advance of move.

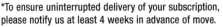